MW01244645

Intermittent Fasting for Women Over 50

A Guide for Beginners in 9 Steps to Eat Clean
and Healthy, Support Hormones and Weight
Loss, with an Intermittent Fasting Lifestyle

Lacy Holland

© Copyright 2020 - All rights reserved.

The content contained within this book may not be reproduced, duplicated or transmitted without direct written permission from the author or the publisher.

Under no circumstances will any blame or legal responsibility be held against the publisher, or author, for any damages, reparation, or monetary loss due to the information contained within this book, either directly or indirectly.

Legal Notice:

This book is copyright protected. It is only for personal use. You cannot amend, distribute, sell, use, quote or paraphrase any part, or the content within this book, without the consent of the author or publisher.

Disclaimer Notice:

Please note the information contained within this document is for educational and entertainment purposes only. All effort has been executed to present accurate, up to date, reliable, complete information. No warranties of any kind are declared or implied. Readers acknowledge that the author is not engaged in the rendering of legal, financial, medical or professional advice. The content within this book has been derived from various sources. Please consult a licensed professional before attempting any techniques outlined in this book.

By reading this document, the reader agrees that under no circumstances is the author responsible for any losses, direct or indirect, that are incurred as a result of the use of the information contained within this document, including, but not limited to, errors, omissions, or inaccuracies.

Table of Contents

Introduction

"Your health is an investment, not an expense!" - Unknown

A s women, we endeavor to know more and to do more. As family women, we pride ourselves on providing and doing the best for those closest to us, but what about us?

If you would have to approach any woman on the street and ask them: "What would you like to change or do more of?" Many would reply: "Look better, feel better, fight my age!" There is no shame in this reply; as mentioned, we always want the best and that means for ourselves as well.

In the 21st century, everyone is selling some form of diet, potion, or lotion to make you look and feel great. It can be overwhelming; however, what if one would have to say there is something, very basic and easy to follow, that will do away with all that is on the market and starts with the items you place into your shopping basket.

No, it is not a diet; it is a lifestyle change. Say hello to intermittent fasting.

What is intermittent fasting you ask, and how does it promise me what it says it is offering, especially if I have, by now, tried almost everything under the sun to curb the weight around my waist and stop the wrinkles tracing lines over my face?

Currently, **intermittent fasting is growing a large following in positively impacting people's overall wellness**. In basic terms, it is the shift between eating and fasting. Though there are no specific foods that should be avoided, healthier options are still (and always) wiser to stick with. The question is more of when food is being eaten, versus not.

We are already fasting while we sleep, so why not increase this time? You could choose to go without eating anything until lunchtime and eating your last meal later than you ordinarily would.

There are a variety of intermittent styles, which this book will go into more detail about. The fast between sleep and eating could be 16 hours or limiting your eating to within six hours a day. This style is called 16:8.

There is also a popular fasting revolution called 5:2, which allows an individual to eat one, calorie-restricted meal of 500 calories two days of the week and return to regular eating the remaining five days of the week.

The eat-stop-eat technique involves eating a proportionate meal at breakfast, lunch, or dinner time and then not eating until the following selected meal time, so technically your fast period is 24 hours.

Intermittent fasting can enhance the loss of weight, help manage and support those who suffer from chronic illness, aid metabolic wellness, and is further said to promote longevity [1]. It can also stabilize blood sugar levels, curb inflammation in the body and remarkably better the brain's ability to deal with memory [2].

Fasting also surprisingly influences how well your heart functions and aids in beating heart disease [3]. Over 47% of Americans have between one and three risk factors related to heart disease [4]. It would seem wise to take the steps needed to prevent or manage it, and fasting is one of the answers to this. Diseases such as cancer may also be prevented too.

Intermittent fasting also causes less muscle loss than standard diets, which is important when considering that with aging comes loss of strength. Furthermore, we all want to live longer, live in the now, and live for what the future brings. Fasting affects our gene expression and how it functions, promoting long life [5].

It can also improve our lives in other areas; think, if you are eating less, the washing of the dishes is less, and that is a plus for any woman in any household. Many times, an individual can find themselves annoyed or even stressed as the prospect of always having to prepare a meal for every mealtime. Not with fasting, and if you are partnered up, it would be wise to ring them into fasting too, not just to support your fasting journey but also to improve their health along the way.

Fasting has been part of our history for many centuries; some religious practices include fasting over important days. Buddhists, Islamists, and Christians fast. Both humans and animals tend to stave off food when ill. Back in the time of the caveman, humans also fasted when access to food was limited. Therefore, there is no recognizable reason why it is not fit to implement into your lifestyle.

No lifestyle change comes easily, but fasting can positively impact all areas of your life; there is proven research into this. There will be days where you find yourself grumpy or hungry or even "*hangry*," a combination of being hungry, which causes you to be angry. As women, our hormones also fluctuate, so there is no reason for you to feel 100% all the time. The only art of intermittent fasting is to stick with it, no matter how many times you stumble.

The time it takes for you to become used to fasting and OK with it could be as little as a few days or weeks; for some, it might take a bit longer, and that is alright too. The same can be said for those expecting immediate results. It all happens differently for us but there are gratifying rewards for all those who choose to fast.

Intermittent fasting does also not have to be a boring affair with food either; it might even encourage you to look at food in a whole new light.

Enjoy the journey, and revel in this new way of life!

Chapter 1: Intermittent Fasting and You

"Every time you eat is an opportunity to nourish your body!"
- Unknown

The age of 50 is no longer what it used to be. In today's world, we are living our best life and seeing the age of 50 only as an extension of our forties. We are living longer, and though statistics regarding some diseases are frightening, we are living healthier lives. We also have access to plenty of information online, which means researching diets, lifestyle changes, and our health are readily available.

Turning 50 opens up a whole new world of possibilities and an opportunity to discover just how we can support ourselves into the next chapter of our life.

Intermittent fasting is one of the answers to many questions on how to live a better, healthier life and curb or prevent diseases that develop with age.

Physical changes are bound to become more noticeable in this time period but you do not have to fear; intermittent fasting allows you to tap into your own body's resources and provide you with a solid foundation in bettering your health and overall wellness.

The practice of intermittent fasting can remarkably change how you age and also understand how capable your body is of recreating itself. I am sure many people would scoff at this statement, but there is truth in this statement. It does not matter where you find yourself in the decade of 50 but read on and see how you have the power to change your life and health through this diet practice.

Cell Regeneration, Longevity, and Immunity

When we begin to age, our body's natural ability to stave off infection and cell regeneration, as linked to age, lessens. In simple terms, it means when we are confronted with an infection, especially gastrointestinal ones, it takes us longer to recover.

When an individual fasts, we are controlling our calorie intake, and scientists have claimed that **a lower intake of calories is directly linked to longevity** [6]. Stem cells are a pivotal part of our health, as they repair any damage occurring internally and externally to the body.

When we fast, it triggers our "*metabolic switch*" that then boosts the level at which our bodies regenerate their cells. These changes on a cellular level are a phenomenal thing to be able to manipulate, and fasting only enhances our ability to do so.

There is still a large amount of research being conducted to further understand the impact metabolic switching has on the body but tests and trials are proving insightful [7]. There is long-standing proof that both our diets and metabolism have profound effects on our susceptibility for illnesses.

When we fast for extended periods, our bodies make use of all the fats and glucose to create ketones, which occur in the liver. These molecules are incredibly beneficial for your brain. For your body to keep functioning during fasting periods, your body naturally rids itself of all the toxins and dead and/or damaged cells.

During this period, energy levels and health levels are boosted. This is beyond helpful for those looking for a cleaner bill of health. Moreover, for those who have damaged cells due to illness like cancer, and receiving treatment like chemotherapy, fasting can recreate a new immune system [8]. A healthier immune system goes hand in hand with longevity and quality of life.

Hormones

Growth Hormone

Our growth hormone is responsible for upping our fats and allowing our bodies to feed on that reserve for energy. **Thanks to the growth hormone, our bodies can sustain bone density and muscle mass**, two very important things worth mentioning in the broader scope of aging. As we age, our growth hormone begins to slow down, leaving us more prone to falls, weakness, joint issues, and muscle aches.

The human growth hormone (HGH) is molded thanks to our pituitary gland and affects how children grow up and it plays just as big a role in adulthood. When the hormone is released, it is only present in the human body for a few short minutes and is then whisked away by the liver to metabolize.

HGH is typically released while we are in a deep sleep and through the long and short of it offsets the effects of insulin.

Just before waking, the human body secretes this hormone and the purpose of this is to begin preparing the body for the day that lies ahead and all the mental and physical demands it will place on us.

The most important meal of the day is not breakfast and the reason for this is because our bodies have already, chemically, ensured that we are set. Generally speaking, we are more inclined to feel hungry later in the day than first thing in the morning.

Fasting is one of the ways to positively up our growth hormone levels, protecting us from aging-related issues. It has been reported that over a five-day cycle of fasting that growth hormones more than doubled [9].

It has been further said that the retention of muscle mass and bone density is four times greater when fasting than it is when restricting calories.

Noradrenaline

Noradrenaline is there to ensure we have enough energy reserves to go and seek more feed. Back in the day of loincloths, hunting, and periods of not eating, you would think that most energy reserves would be depleted, that there would be no will power to want to get up on an empty stomach and physically go and hunt for your next meal. Noradrenaline is there to make sure that even hungry, we have the power to do so [10].

Our **metabolic rate is increased by 3.6% if we fast** for 48 hours. Fasting over two days does not cause our metabolic system to shut off; it can do the exact opposite.

Fasting changes up where it is getting its energy reserves from, instead of burning up the sugars it turns to fat. The great news is that the level at which our metabolic rate rests is thus increased.

The fat found in our bodies can be thought of as rich energy reserves, which protect us from starving. In today's world, there is very little chance of that happening, so the fat is not needed. Intermittent fasting is how we bypass the sugar and tap into the stored fat.

Electrolytes

As mentioned, as we live in the 21st century with minimal chances of going hungry for long and we have a very small likelihood of developing a nutrient deficiency. The fact that our bodies hoard is enough to keep us going for quite a while.

Potassium levels may drop but research has shown that it did not drop low enough to be detrimental to your health and leaves little to no effect on the body.

All other important nutrients such as calcium, phosphorus, and magnesium hold steady during fasting, which is good news for ladies over 50s. Over 90% of the calcium and phosphorus in our bodies stems from our bones.

If you are at all concerned about the levels of minerals in your body, **supplements are a natural way to help support the body**. With any taking of medication, holistic or not, ensure you discuss this with your doctor first.

Insulin

Research has indicated that **fasting is one of the main ways in which to lower insulin** levels. All types of food, healthy and unhealthy increase the levels of insulin in our bodies, therefore it makes common sense, deny all foods and decrease that level.

Fasts for 24 to 36 hours have shown to reduce the insulin level whereas fasts that last longer can even more rapidly lower the insulin. Alternate day fasting is also a recommended way in which to control these levels.

There are a lot of diets we can pick and choose from, all offering weight loss miracles. They do address dropping insulin levels by providing diets that control high insulin producing foods. It does, however, not address the problem of insulin resistance in the body. Fasting is there to not only lower insulin levels but also manage insulin resistance, a pivotal part of long-term weight loss [11].

Extra water and salt are stored in the body; by decreasing the levels of insulin, we are helping support the body by getting rid of these elements. Salt and water can build up in the kidneys because of insulin.

Lowering insulin resistance further allows the body to regulate blood sugar levels and provide protection against developing type 2 diabetes. The main job of insulin is to manage blood sugar levels. The human body also detests having too much of it floating around, even though we use it for energy.

If we eat a diet rich in carbohydrates, the sugar levels rise within our bodies. The pancreas begins pumping out insulin. If the small, humble organ begins to feel overwhelmed by a diet fueled with sugars and carbs, it churns out more insulin. Insulin also controls the fat within our bodies; what it does with the fat cells is it removes them and stores them away from your blood. It is partly thanks to the insulin that causes us to be overweight. The more there is of it, the more fat it is stashing away, running you the risk of potentially developing cancer too.

If we condition our bodies in such a manner to accept the large amounts of insulin, we produce the cells become resistant towards it. Blood sugar levels are higher than average and stay this way, translating to developing type 2 diabetes. As of 2015, it was reported by the World Health Organization that over 400 million people across the world suffered from this disease. [12].

Diabetes

The most common form of diabetes is type 2 diabetes. It does not have to be a death sentence and can be controlled through what we put into our bodies. When we age, we become more susceptible to developing this illness. Men, more so than women. If your weight is located more around your middle than anywhere else, then it would be wise to seriously look at changing your eating habits for the better.

Of the 400 million individuals who have type 2 diabetes worldwide, 29.1 million are American, and a further 8.1 million are said to be unaware that they have it. Nearly 1.5 million cases are reported annually in the United States alone.

Many people also have pre-diabetes; one out of three are usually diagnosed. A further nine out of ten won't even know they have it either.

Almost 26% of adults over the age of 65 have been diagnosed with diabetes. The largest age group is made up of those between the ages of 40 and 59.

Factors that determine if you are at risk are:

- Bad diet
- Limited physical activity
- Genetics
- Age
- Weight distributed around your middle, stomach area

Issues that arise with those who have type 2 diabetes include:

- Hypertension
- Stroke
- Amputations
- Disease within the kidneys
- Skin-related problems
- Eye trouble
- Heart disease
- Depression
- Dental trouble

Fasting and following a regular exercise program are the best ways in which you can avoid developing the disease, or if you have been diagnosed, managing the illness.

Following up with your doctor is also a wise decision to make, and keeping an eye on your bloodwork, blood pressure, cholesterol, and sugar levels is also a wise move.

The management of your weight is also crucial in staving off the illness, thus exercising and fasting go hand in hand with helping you achieve weight loss.

Heart Health

There is a considerable amount of research being done with regard to heart health and the impact that intermittent fasting has on it. Results look promising and show that intermittent fasting can be one of the main tools we could utilize to reduce our risk of heart disease.

One of the main reasons why people show better health when fasting is because they practice a level of control when it comes to diet and exercise. This way of living tends to spill over into their regular ways of eating, even on days where they are not fasting. Both diet and exercise prove yet again to be vital when avoiding any form of illness [13].

Fasting also controls your blood-sugar and cholesterol levels, both factors which impact your likelihood of developing heart disease or suffering from a heart attack. Fasting decreases the level of "bad" cholesterol—lipoprotein—in your bloodstream and manages how our bodies metabolize sugar.

By controlling these two elements, it helps us avoid developing type 2 diabetes and obesity, both of which are two contributing factors when mentioning heart disease.

Science goes on to mention that it controls our blood pressure and reduces our insulin resistance. Further research conducted has shown that fasters have a 45% lesser rate of mortality than non-fasters. Fasters have also shown to have a 71% lesser rate of developing heart disease and related illnesses [14].

Circadian Rhythm

What is the circadian rhythm and how does it affect you? **Circadian rhythm is the process that occurs internally within your body to regulate your sleep and wake cycles.** This cycle repeats every 24 hours.

Over the centuries, our bodies have become used to eating during the day and sleeping at night. However, humans have begun to blur this rhythm by eating way past the time the sun goes down. Those people who eat late at night have shown to be more susceptible to obesity and developing type 2 diabetes [15].

Intermittent fasting allows us to finish meals earlier on in the day and extends the period of which our bodies aren't receiving food; this factors in your sleep period where food is not being consumed either [16].

Aligning our diet with the circadian rhythm is beneficial for long-term health and avoiding disease.

Though results may vary from individual to individual, the following benefits may also be experienced:

- Better sleeping at night; fewer periods of waking
- Less sugar cravings when awake
- Less caffeine cravings during the day
- Higher energy levels
- Weight loss
- Less water retention and swelling
- Less body and joint pain
- Decreased appetite

Circadian rhythms can affect hormonal changes, sleep patterns, body temperature, and eating habits, so it makes sense to align yourself with the rhythm of your body [17].

When this rhythm becomes inconsistent, it can lead to other health-related issues such as insomnia, heart disease, diabetes, depression, and obesity.

Autophagy

Autophagy is designed to allow the body to toss out all the damaged or dead cells that the body no longer needs and replace them with stronger, healthier cells that will then continue to benefit the body.

To harness autophagy, intermittent fasting comes highly recommended [18]. To understand the dynamics of it, see it like this: when we eat, insulin goes up and glucagon goes down; when we do not eat, insulin goes down and glucagon goes up. Glucagon is an important hormone in the body; the higher it is, the faster it can stimulate autophagy from taking place within the body.

Cell repair and renewal is the answer to slower aging and fighting disease [19]. The healthier the cells and the more cells within our bodies, the healthier we are.

Remember low autophagy levels can be detrimental to our health, the same way high levels of it can pose a risk. There has to be an even balance mastered and that is eating and not eating, as well as avoiding a life of contestant calorie-restricted diets.

Cancer

Research has further indicated that intermittent fasting can prevent cancer and can support those who are undergoing cancer treatment.

The reason that intermittent fasting can aid in the prevention of cancer is that it has been known to lower insulin resistance and curb inflammation in the body. Both triggers can cause cancer to form in the body.

For those who are currently undergoing chemotherapy, it has been said that intermittent fasting might aid the cells within the body to become more susceptible to chemotherapy and fight the cancer that is already within the body.

Controlling our blood sugar levels through intermittent fasting and lowering our insulin resistance is said to restrict the ability of cancers to grow [20].

As type 2 diabetes and obesity are risk factors for heart disease, they are also to risk factors for cancer.

Intermittent fasting lowers the level of toxicities in the human body, which has been said to support the outcome of those undergoing chemotherapy.

Studies conducted in 2016 showed that intermittent fasting, along with chemotherapy treatment, slowed the development of skin and breast cancer [21]. Intermittent fasting protects the cells while undergoing treatment and encourages the growth of stem cells in the body.

Weight Loss

In simple terms, **intermittent fasting allows the body to tap into its fat stores** for energy, resulting in weight loss.

Excess fat is burnt to sustain the body in the periods that we are fasting.

To further understand the dynamics of weight loss and intermittent fasting, know that when we eat, in general, we are adding more energy to the body than what is required at that time, leaving the body to metabolize a portion and store a portion. When you fast, you metabolize what you have eaten and then progress to metabolizing your fat reserves to sustain you till the end of the day.

By shortening the window in which we eat means that during the periods we aren't eating our body has to look somewhere for energy, and intermittent fasting guides it to its reserves, so bye-bye fat [22].

Insulin levels are influenced by intermittent fasting, which lowers it. The signals sent to the body tell it to look for energy in other places as it is no longer coming from food.

Weight gain occurs as we have kept the body in a feeding state from sunup to sundown, not allowing the body to tap into its reserves, which it should be doing regularly.

Weight loss comes in when we spend time in the non-fed state, so welcome intermittent fasting, which places our bodies into this period.

Intermittent fasting also boosts your resting metabolic rate, meaning when you are not eating, you are still burning energy higher than what you would before fasting.

Moods

Evidence suggest that diets high in sugar, processed foods, and fat disturb the natural occurring flora within the gut and interfere with the brain-gut axis; in simple terms, it means that bad eating can affect our moods and eating an unhealthy diet very well may cause depression, anxiety, stress, mood swings, and irritability. A bad diet has also been known to aggravate these mental problems if you do generally suffer from them [23].

Diets rich in healthy foods and to practice a level of control when it comes to sugars, fats, and processed food indicate that it can reduce these issues.

It has been further noted that following intermittent fasting or other calorie-controlled, whole-food rich diets may very well improve these mental ailments. Furthermore, diets such as intermittent fasting and calorie-controlled diets are said to further support and boost the effects of antidepressants in patients who use the medication to treat mental illness.

Mental illness such as anxiety is the most prevalent mental illness in America. Over 40 million adults are affected. Sadly, only 36.9% receive treatment for the disorder [24].

Brain Health

The brain is probably the most complex and intriguing organ in the world. Our brains are so powerful and allow us to do a variety of tasks, from reading, writing, signing, sorting through complex puzzles, math, building items, and experiencing emotions, to name a few.

It would seem important to only want to preserve and protect it by all means as it promotes our overall health and quality of life.

Science suggests that the human brain functions far better while in its fasting state than a non-fasting state.

Memory, alertness, and cognitive abilities are remarkably improved during a fasting state than when we are eating [25].

When we age, our cognitive decline becomes more apparent; it is something that many people will struggle with. Memory also tends to fade and thinking patterns are also slow.

Basic brain puzzles are a good way to improve and exercise your brain. Along with fasting, you have a chance at protecting and preserving your brain's ability. Fasting may fight off diseases such as memory loss, dementia, and Alzheimer's.

Over 5.8 million Americans live with Alzheimer's; it is a terrible disease that interferes with memory, changes a person's mood, and meddles with the thinking process [26].

If diagnosed with dementia or Alzheimer's, there is no cure but intermittent fasting may help prevent the illness or be able to delay it.

Tests, currently underway on lab rats and mice, indicate that fasting lessens cognitive decline and helps aid in the management of Alzheimer's symptoms. Studies have begun to move to humans in hope that intermittent fasting might be the answer in preventing and curing specific diseases [27].

Energy Levels

Many would think that intermittent fasting would impact our energy levels in a bad way. Generally, on a regular day of eating, our blood sugar levels go up and down, interfering with how we feel in the energy department. When we feel even a small inkling of being hungry, we tend to go look for something to satisfy the feeling. When the body has taken what it needs after eating, our energy levels drop. When this happens, the body revs itself up again and says you need food. The stress that the body is then placed under during this to-and-fro reduces our metabolic rate too.

When you fast, the fat that is consumed is first sent to the liver before anything else happens to it and before it begins releasing energy. As this process happens gradually, especially when fasting, our energy levels are maintained throughout the day.

We have more energy and we are cognitively sharper during this period.

The switch to intermittent fasting is a gradual one that your body will have to get used to, so do not expect to have bundles of energy in the initial stages. **Your body has to be trained on how to fast; the more you fast, the more your body adapts** and the more energy it can provide you with [28].

The hormone ghrelin, responsible for making us feel hungry, becomes better controlled through fasting, so it is less inclined to flare up and demand food, leaving you less hungry and, in turn, ups your energy levels.

Skin Health

Diet has a profound effect on the clarity of and health of our skin, the largest organ of the body.

Inflammatory diseases can wreak havoc on the human body and their symptoms can be manageable to severe. Common inflammatory issues are eczema and acne.

These two inflammatory conditions can cause unsightly marks and you do not have to be a particular age to develop it; these conditions can also occur much later on in life too. These marks can cause many people to become self-conscious and hide away from the public eye.

The body has strong ties to the gut. Foods can cause inflammation throughout the body. It makes sense that a calorie-controlled diet such as intermittent fasting, which should be rich in nutritious foods and low in sugar, can help support those who have these conditions or even prevent them.

Intermittent fasting fuels the antioxidants within our bodies, resulting in better-looking skin, with fewer wrinkles and age spots [29].

It is important that when fasting to ensure you are eating the best foods for your health that cater to all your nutritional requirements.

Intermittent Fasting and You Round-Up

- It can beat cancer.
- It helps avoid heart-related diseases and suffering from a stroke or heart attack.
- It can be used to treat and prevent inflammation within the body.
- Boosts your energy levels.
- It can prevent you from developing Alzheimer's, cognitive decline, and dementia, and IF provides support for those who have already been diagnosed.
- Say hello to longevity.
- Control circadian rhythms; prevent diabetes and obesity.
- Boosts autophagy, the management of cells needed for improved health.

Thanks for choosing this book, make sure to leave a short review on Amazon if you enjoy it. I'd really love to hear your thoughts.

Chapter 2: Your Body at 50

"I never think about age. I believe your age is totally how you feel. I've seen women of 35 who are old and people of 75 who are young. As long as I look after myself physically, mentally and emotionally, I will stay young." - Joan Collins

With age comes wisdom, but it also comes with a few other not so pleasant changes, which for many women, might be hard to accept. Aging gracefully is what the majority hope for and to ease aging symptoms, which become more recognizable and can be felt in certain areas of the body.

The beauty is that, yes, we age, but in modern times, we have a world of opportunity to curb these changes with lotions, potions, eating programs, and exercise regimes. People who are over the age of 50 are living their best life and instead of winding down, are venturing out and exploring what the world has to offer.

Women will always be conscious of the way they look; it's part of who we are. It would be wise to understand how your body changes from the time you hit 50. To become aware of these changes will go a long way in you taking preventative measures to control them and improve your health and wellness.

When we hit 50, things begin to slow down, such as our metabolic function, blood flow, and healing [30]. Genes and how we did and currently look after our bodies will also determine how aging affects us.

Aging does not need to be all doom and gloom; no, you can take measures to help support you and your body through the process and effects. Intermittent fasting and exercise are a couple of ways in which this can be done.

Bladder Control

If you are a woman who has borne children, then more than likely your bladder would be one of the things on the list that would be the most impacted by age. Muscle decline and menopause are a few reasons why a "leaky" bladder can occur too.

The best method to curb this is to practice Kegel exercises. How you do this is very simple: simply tighten your pelvic muscles and vaginal area as if you were "*pinching*." It is important to keep your legs, stomach, and buttocks relaxed and do not hold your breath while clenching. Do three sets of 10, or clench, count for three seconds, release, and clench again for three seconds; do this 10 times over. Practice in the comfort of your bedroom or bathroom, also not while you are urinating.

Do these exercises every day; they will strengthen the muscles in that area and support your bladder.

Also, it is advised to avoid:

- Alcohol
- Coffee
- Tea

Brain Health

Mental health can take a knock at 55. The best way to improve your brain health is by adjusting your diet and that is why intermittent fasting is considered one of the best ways to promote better brain health.

Eat plenty of:

- Leafy-green vegetables
- Fresh fruit
- Cook with extra-virgin olive oil
- Eat a rich diet of whole-grains

Mental Health

Menopause comes with a list of nagging symptoms; one of them can be your mental health, and because of hormonal changes, our moods can fluctuate and this may lead to depression. The number one strategy to invest in is to get moving; leading a sedentary life does no good for positive thinking and mental health.

Try these activities to beat depression:

- Swimming
- Yoga
- Art classes
- Volunteer work
- Meditation

Eat the following to help support your mental health.

- Salmon
- Trout
- Prawns

In particular, these foods contain docosahexaenoic acid (DHA), super-foods for your brain, which can beat anxiety and boost memory function.

Hormonal Health

As we age, our estrogen levels begin to dwindle. Their primary function is to manage the health of the reproductive system and keep the blood supply up.

Everything we put into our bodies can in some way, shape, and form impact your hormonal balance, and at a stage in your life where there are big changes in this department, it is important to know what you can do to improve your mood and the way you feel and, of course, avoid the nasty, gritty things that hamper you from feeling like you are 21 again. The guide below falls in-line with intermittent fasting because eating and hormones go hand in hand and allow you to balance your hormones.

Low levels of estrogen can cause:

- Vaginal dryness
- Night sweats
- Dry skin
- Bad memory
- Heart palpitations
- Low libido levels
- Inability to sleep
- Depression

Try adding the following to your diet:

- Sesame seeds
- Chickpeas
- All legumes

- Grass-fed and organic meats, at least three times a week
- Apples
- Cherries
- Celery
- Carrots
- Plums
- Pomegranate
- Tomatoes
- Cucumber
- Dates
- Papaya

Stay away from:

- Soy products
- Processed foods

Hair and Skin Changes

Skin becomes less elastic and can become dry. Hair also becomes grey. Keep up the care of your skin by wearing sunscreen and a hat when outdoors. Research has confirmed that diet can remarkably impact the appearance of our skin and fight off fine lines and wrinkles.

The following foods can remarkably change the appearance of your skin:

- Blueberries
- Broccoli
- Watercress
- Red bell peppers
- Spinach
- All nuts

Immunity

After 50, our body is less inclined to fight off infections and diseases and we are more susceptible to falling ill. This is down to the fact that the cells produced to fight infections are not created so quickly as when we were younger.

It is important to include the following to your diet:

- Garlic
- Ginger
- Citrus fruits
- Berry fruits
- Bell peppers
- Yogurt

Metabolism and Weight Changes

Just because things are slowing down does not mean we should panic. When hitting the 50 mark, women can find it harder to shed the weight than before, and this is completely normal and one of the many things that change with age.

For women, most of the fat we gain after 50 tends to sit around our middles. This is partially thanks to insulin resistance, which increases with age. As the cells in our bodies struggle with absorbing glucose, it leads to increased sugar levels, which can further contribute to developing type 2 diabetes.

Stay away from:

- Refined carbohydrates
- White flours
- Sugar
- Bread

- Candy

Say yes to:

- Lean protein
- Fresh fruits and vegetables
- Whole-grain and products

By 50, our metabolism begins to function 15% less than when we were younger. This begins to happen already in our 30s.

Heart Health

After 50, our risks of heart-related disease go up and the likelihood of suffering a heart attack increases too. Exercise is one of the ways, along with a strict diet, that can control this outcome. You should exercise for 30 minutes a day, every day.

Your Body at 50 Round-Up

- Choose to eat as organically as you can.
- Opt for organically produced and created home and beauty products.
- Stay away from canned foods or those wrapped in plastic.
- Eat a diet that is filled with the right things that boost your liver function and provide protection for your body such as asparagus, garlic, chives, pears, pumpkin, and cauliflower.
- Wash fruits and vegetables before consumption.
- Wear sunscreen every day, even in the winter.
- Keep your blood sugar levels under control.
- Monitor your blood pressure.
- Stop smoking.

- Drink a cup of chamomile tea before bedtime.
- Get good a good night's rest.

Chapter 3: What Fast Is Best?

"Let your food be your medicine." - Hippocrates

What Fast Is Best?

There are numerous types of intermittent fasting regimes that are available for you to follow, which is great news for finding the most suitable one for you and being able to fit it into your current lifestyle [31].

Results vary from one person to another, so the best recommendation is to sample the various types of fasting and find one that suits you. Luckily, **fasting requires minimal effort** in having to rush off and buy unique ingredients; all you have to do is eat less that is in your pantry than what you originally did.

Always consult with a doctor before undertaking any change of eating and if you have a pre-existing medical condition or taking medication.

For those who would like to fast but are unsure how to **proceed, seeking the help of a dietician may help you pursue your fasting journey**, as these professionals are equipped to help set out a plan for you to follow with meals included, which could ease you into this lifestyle change.

Be sure to always eat a balanced meal on fasting and non-fasting days to give your body the best chance of functioning and promoting your overall wellness.

Here are several fasting styles to help you on your way.

Warrior Diet

This diet is probably the most drastic form of fasting as the window in which a person consumes food is very small; think four hours of eating, and 20 hours of no eating. During the window of eating, only raw fruits, vegetables, and lean proteins are consumed, followed by a balanced meal in the evening.

This type of fasting is better recommended for people who have already practiced a variety of other fasts or have chosen to extend the hours of their fasting.

The concept of this way of eating is that it is said that people are nocturnal eaters. When we eat at night, our body is said to align itself to our cardiac rhythms and steady our heart-rate.

The warrior diet offers a far more rigid way of eating and it is expected that you stick to the hours of eating and not eating. Some find this hard to adapt to; therefore, it is for the more advanced faster who is conscious of what to eat and when to eat. While following this fasting method, ensure no nutrients such as fiber are excluded from your diet.

24-Hour Fast

Some people readily adjust to this way of eating. **The 24-hour diet is exactly that: no eating for 24 hours** and applying it once or twice a week.

So, a fast will be from breakfast to breakfast, lunch to lunch, or dinner to dinner.

This type of fasting is also considered rather drastic for beginners and is advised for the more advanced faster who wishes to extend their period of fasting.

Like all fasting diets, you are allowed to drink water, black tea and coffee, and bone broth.

The guidelines of fasting are important to stick with and to not deviate from. A return to normal eating should happen the day after the 24-hour fast and should not be followed by another 24-hour fast.

This way of eating may come with some uncomfortable feelings such as hunger, tiredness, and headaches. Do make note that this type of eating does require commitment and that like all eating regimes, your body will adapt and the symptoms will pass.

On-Off Eating

This way of eating and fasting has already been practiced by yourself and countless other people across the world; you just weren't aware it was part of a fasting program. **The on-off way of eating is simple; you might choose to skip breakfast and continue with regular eating come lunchtime.** You could choose to eat breakfast, skip lunch, and eat dinner.

Whenever you do eat a meal, it is important to still stick to the rules of eating healthier options and staying away from sugar, processed foods, and fats.

The idea is simple: you eat only when hungry and not because of any other reason such as boredom. This is an easy program to follow and good for those who wish to start their fasting journey slowly and gradually before moving onto more serious ways of fasting.

12-Hour fast

The **12-hour fast is when 12 hours pass between you eating anything.** It is easy to adapt to and a very common way of fasting. The concept is that you eat breakfast, say for example, at seven in the morning, and then only eat again at seven in the evening.

The portion control remains at 500 calories on these days and you fast on two days of the week, and not consecutively. It has been said that if you fast for between 10 and 16 hours a day, our body is inclined to begin to use its fat stores for energy, thus fueling weight loss.

As an alternative, you could choose to finish a meal at seven in the evening, go to bed and eat your next meal at seven in the morning; thus, your fasting period occurred while you were sleeping.

This is a good option for those who are serious about weight loss and who can manage the time between meals.

16:8 Method

Also commonly referred to as the Leangains Diet or 14:10 from women. This type of **fasting schedule is one of the** most **popular ways of fasting** and comes highly recommended for beginners and those looking to shed the pounds.

A person will fast for 16 hours a day and be left with a window period for eating that will last eight hours. For women, you can decrease the fasting window to 14 hours and eating window to 10 hours; the reason for this is to factor in our hormones versus men.

Individuals will eat their last meal at seven or eight in the evening, skip breakfast and then go onto eating at midday. The calories are controlled to 500 for women and there are regular snacking periods in the eight-hour eating window, which helps get you to the end of your day and fast.

A one-week fasting plan is mentioned in chapter 7 for you to use as a guideline.

5:2 Fasting

For beginners, this style should be attempted first or the 14:10 method. The reason being is that it is simple to follow and easy to apply to your lifestyle.

The concept is simple: eat regularly for five days and on two, non-consecutive days, you fast, eating only 500 calories on these days.

The reason for its success and easy adaptability is because you are only giving up two days of your week to eat in a restricted manner and returning to your normal, regular eating pattern on your non-fasting days.

The diet is also recommended for those seeking to lose weight and it helps prevent heart disease. This diet is beneficial for overall heart health and has been known to influence insulin levels for the better.

Reports suggest that people who follow this plan can seek to lose 11 pounds over 12 weeks.

A basic schedule of three fasting patterns is mentioned in chapter 7 for you to apply if you feel that this type of fasting method is best suited to your current lifestyle.

When Fasting Should Be Avoided

On all accounts, fasting is becoming one of the fastest eating trends and with good reason. However, like many undertakings, it does come with a certain amount of risk and it should be noted that women should not pursue this lifestyle change if they represent one or more of these:

- Suffer from insomnia
- Have an eating disorder or have a history of eating disorders
- Diagnoses with chronic stress
- Pregnant
- Breastfeeding
- Underweight

Consult your doctor if you suffer from one or more of the below mentioned before pursuing too fast:

- Diabetes
- Low blood pressure
- Take chronic medication for a medical condition
- Suffer from blood sugar irregularities

Contraindications

Chronic Stress

Chronic stress can be aggravated when undertaking a fast, as fasting may trigger the stress hormone, which is counterintuitive to your well-being.

Pre- or Post-Surgery

If you are going to undergo a fairly large operation or are in the recovery stages of an operation, it would be unwise to pursue fasting. Your body needs all it can to help it through the stress of surgery and the after-effects it has on the body. Your body uses more nutrients, vitamins, and minerals during recovery and needs as many reserves as possible to restore it to what it was.

Wintertime Effects

It is advised that you fast during the spring and summer months; the reasoning behind this is that fasting during winter may cause the body to store what it is fed rather than to burn it. The colder it is, the more our bodies burn calories to keep it warm. Fasting through winter can also cause nutrient deficiencies and other related ailments.

Common Fasting Mistakes

We all like to see results when we have worked hard at something, including the relationship most women have with the bathroom scale. Sometimes, when the day finally arrives to stand on the scale, we see little to no changes, or we see a higher weight than what we initially recorded when the choice was made to begin fasting.

Many mistakes to be corrected, restoring what fasting was meant to achieve. The following mistakes are common and easy to make but are simple to fix.

Exercising to Hard

If you used to exercise and put a lot of effort in working out, then there should not be any reason that your body would be negatively impacted, nor the scale.

For those who decided to pair fasting with exercising for the first time, you might want to **start with a very light exercise regime** instead of going at it like a bodybuilder. It is recommended that you do allow periods of recovery when exercising; therefore, it is a wise decision to get to bed early and skip your workout on the days that you do fast or consider lightening your exercise on your fasting days and lessening the time you exercise.

Most importantly, get the sleep you need. This time is when the body can restore itself and build reserves for tackling the following day. You should be getting anything from between seven to nine hours of sleep a night; women would be happy to hear that sleep reins in our moods too!

You Are Not Staying Hydrated

Even though we are eating plenty of nutrient-rich fruits and vegetables, however, during the periods between meals or fasts, you should be staying hydrated by drinking enough water. **For those who struggle with their hunger, drinking bone broth comes highly recommended** and restores important electrolytes, leaving you less inclined to feel nauseous or light-headed.

Fasting More Than Recommended

When you have selected the fast of your choosing, the idea is to **stick to it and its rules**. Deviating from this could end up making you feel worse and hamper your progress. You might be inclined to think that more of a better way of life is good for you, but it can increase stress hormones, such as cortisol, which is bad for you and can cause you to binge eat on the days that you are not fasting because your body does not feel satisfied.

Start any fasting regime slowly and consciously; start with fasting one to two days a week, and depending on your fast, begin with 12 hours at a time. You could choose to add more days or hours as you become more comfortable with the concept.

You Are Not Stocking Up on the Right Foods

It is a common mistake to make when you are fasting as you are consuming fewer calories; therefore, the calories that we are allowed to consume should be made of healthy foods that are rich in vitamins. Nutrient deficiencies can arise when calories are restricted. **Eat avocados, lean proteins, nuts, and seeds** to make sure this does not occur and help support your blood sugar levels.

Make sure your intake of healthy, unprocessed foods remains consistent throughout the days that you fast and on the days that you do not. Food empty of nutrients and vitamins will negatively impact your body during the fasting period. As you are eating less on the fasting days, it is pivotal that you eat the best for your overall health.

You Are Not Eating Enough

Above mentions that you might very well be stocking up on the wrong foods but the same can be said for those who are restricting their calories to even less than the 500 on fasting days. The same way overeating on these days won't provide results, undereating will also hamper them. **Make sure you eat as close to 500 calories as possible** and no less.

Pick the Right Plan

Undertaking any diet is filled with hits and misses; the same can be said for the variety of intermittent fasting programs there are available. If you find that one type of intermittent fasting plan does not work for you, do not give up. Simply try another fasting program instead. You might find more success with it.

We are all built and engineered differently: what works for one person need not be the same with regard to your own body.

Fasting Round-Up

- Eat enough food during your fasting days.
- Eat the right foods on your fast days and regular days.
- Get rest.
- Exercise, but do not overdo it.
- Pick the plan that is right for you and your body.
- Eat nutrient-rich foods.
- Keep up your fluids throughout the day.
- If you have a medical condition, see a doctor before fasting.
- Listen to your body, and adapt where necessary.

- Stick to the rules and guidelines of your particular fast of choice.
- Results vary from one person to another; be patient.

Chapter 4: How to Plan Intermittent Fasting

"Winning and losing isn't everything. Sometimes the journey is as important as the outcome." - Alex Morgan

Once you have established the type of intermittent fasting plan that best suits you, you can finally put the plan into action. There is no time like the present and it is wise to begin fasting as soon as you can, giving you less time to procrastinate about all the when, what and ifs.

Setting up a basic plan of action is simple when it comes to fasting. Our pantries and refrigerators also do not need to be overpopulated with rare and expensive ingredients. Fasting is simple and it can be done, more than likely, with the items you already have stored in your kitchen cupboards.

Creating a plan of action is the sure-fire way in which to implement this new lifestyle change. It will help you to track your progress and, in the long term, help you manage and maintain your weight loss and health.

A plan allows you to visually see the work you are putting into fasting and to track results. Plus, it will leave you feeling less frazzled when it comes to your fast day and you are unsure of what meals you will be eating and at what times.

Take gradual steps and, eventually, you will be able to master the art of fasting and adapting it into your current lifestyle.

How to Plan

Step One - Create a Monthly Calendar

On a calendar, highlight the days on which you wish to fast, depending on the type of fast you have committed yourself to. Record a start and end time on your fasting days so you know in the days leading up to your fast day what time you plan to begin and finish.

Tick off your days; this will keep you motivated and on track!

Step Two - Record Your Findings

Create a journal for your fasting journey. One or two days before the time, undertake to do your measurements. Weigh yourself first thing in the morning, after you have gone to the restroom and before breakfast. Also, do not weigh yourself wearing heavy items as they may affect the outcome of the scale.

Measure your height as this figure is related to your BMI (body mass index) result.

Record the measurements around your hips and stomach area, if you wish, you can also measure your upper thighs and arms.

Take a photo of yourself and place it into the journal too; this is not to discourage you but to keep you focused on why you began this journey.

Jot down all of these findings and update them weekly in the journal.

A journal is also the perfect way to express how you are feeling and, of course, what you are most thankful for. **A journal is an important way in which to track not just the physical aspects of the diet but also the mental aspects too.** Never undertake to doubt yourself; your journal should be a safe space for you to congratulate and to motivate yourself. Leave all the negative thoughts at the door!

Step Three - Plan Your Meals

The easiest way to stick to any eating program is to **plan your meals**; 500 calorie meals tend to be simple and easy to create but there are also many other more complex recipes for those who wish to spice things up. Who knows, perhaps you stumble across a meal you wish to eat outside of your fasting days.

It is advised that you **prepare your meals the day before** your fast days; doing this helps you stay committed to the fast and limits food wastage.

Initially, and in the first few weeks, it is suggested that you **keep your meal preparation and recipes simple**, so as not to overcomplicate the whole process. This also allows you to get used to counting your calories and knowing which foods work to keep you fuller versus those that left you feeling hungrier earlier than later.

Be sure to include your meal plan in your journal and on your calendar.

Step Four - Reward Yourself

On the days where you may return to normal eating, **it is important to reward yourself**. A small reward goes a long way in reminding yourself and your brain that what you are doing has merit and that it should be noticed.

A reward should cater to one of our primal needs; these needs include:

- Self-actualization
- Safety needs
- Social needs
- Esteem needs
- Physiological needs such as food, water, air, clothing, and shelter

Have a block of chocolate, or buy yourself a new item of clothing; do anything that makes your heart happy!

Step Five - Curb Hunger Pains

Initially, you will feel more discomfort when hungry but these feelings will pass. If you do find yourself craving something, **sip on black tea or coffee** to help you through your day. Coffee is known to alleviate the feelings of being hungry; if you must add sweetener, do so at your discretion. Know that some sweeteners can cause the opposite effect and make you feel hungry.

Step Six - Stay Busy

Keeping busy means that the mind does not have time to dwell on your current state of affairs, especially if you find yourself reaching for a snack bar or cookie.

It is also wise to be implementing some sort of physical activity, even on your fasting days. **A 20-minute walk before ending your fasting period will do wonders** to help you reach the final stages of the fasting period. It can also uplift your mood when you are feeling frustrated or tense.

Step Seven - Practice Mindful Eating

As mentioned, we are inclined to eat for all sorts of reasons; happy, sad, it does not matter. The problem is that these feelings related to food become habitual, so we aren't really hungry but because we feel good or even off, we seek to tuck into something delicious.

The art of **eating mindfully is to not allow these habits to master your life**. The concept is simple: teach yourself to look at something, for instance, a piece of cake and think, "Do I really need it or do I want it for other reasons?" You could decide to have a bite or two and leave the rest, but you may be less inclined to eat the whole slice (or whole cake) if you think mindfully about it.

The art of mindful eating is to revel in the food placed before you. Pay attention to the colors, textures, and tastes. Savor each bite, even when eating an apple.

Your brain gradually begins to rewire itself when it comes to food and when it needs or wants something.

Practice mindful eating by:

- Pay attention to where your food comes from.
- **Listen to what your body is telling you**; stop eating when you are full.
- Only eat when your body signals you to do so; when your stomach growls or if you feel faint or if your energy levels are low.

- Pay attention to what is both healthy and unhealthy for us.
- Consider the environmental impact our food choices make.
- Every time you take a bite of your meal, set your cutlery down.

Step Eight - Practice Portion Control

Controlling portion sizes can be difficult for most; society has also regulated us to what we think is the size of an average portion should be and we have access to supersizing meals too, which does not help those struggling in the weight department. In 1961, Americans consumed 2,880 calories per day; by 2017, they were consuming 3,600 calories, which is a 34% increase and an unhealthy one at that.

To help you navigate how to better portion your food, consider trying the following: when dishing up your food, try the following trick. Half of your plate should consist of healthy fruits and/or vegetables, one quarter should be made up of your starches such as potatoes, rice, or pasta, and the remaining quarter should be made up of lean meats or seafood.

Alternatively, try the following:

- Dish up onto a smaller plate or into a smaller bowl.
- Say no to upsizing a meal if offered.
- Buy the smaller version of the product if available, or divide the servings equally into packets.
- Eat half a meal at the restaurant and take the remaining half to enjoy the following day instead.
- Go to bed early; it will stop any after-dinner eating.

Step Nine - Get Tech Savvy

Modern-day society has plenty to offer us in terms of the apps we can use to help determine the steps we take, the calories we burn, the calories found in our foods, as well as research, information, and motivation for lifestyle changes, especially diets and exercise. The list is endless. There are many apps on the market currently that can help you track your progress with regards to fasting.

The best intermittent fasting apps of currently (at the time of writing), and in no particular order are:

- Zero
- FastHabit
- BodyFast
- Fastient
- Vora
- Ate Food Diary
- Life Fasting Tracker

Make use of your mobile device to set reminders for yourself of when to eat, what to eat, and when your fast days are. It works especially well when using it to set reminders for when you should drink water, particularly for those who find it hard to keep their fluids up.

Making the Change

Understand that intermittent fasting is not a diet; it is a lifestyle, an eating plan that you are in control of and one that is easy to perfect. Before you know it, fasting will become second nature.

When to Start?

Begin today, not tomorrow or after a particular event or gathering. Once you have picked the fast that best suits you, begin with it immediately. Never hold off until a specific day; once you begin, you will gain momentum and it will become something that is part of your day, like many other things that fill up your day. No sweat there!

Measure Your Eating

Three days before you fast, it would be wise to begin to lessen the amount of food you are eating or dishing up less. This helps your body begin to get used to the idea that it doesn't need a whole bowl of food to get what it needs nor to feel full.

Keep up Your Exercise Plan

If you have a pre-existing exercise regime, do not alter it anyway. Simply carry on the way you were before fasting. If you are new to exercising, begin with short walks now and again, extending the time you walk. For example, take a five-minute walk, and the next day, change the time to 10 minutes of walking.

Stop, Start, Stop

Fast for a period of hours, and then eat all your calories during a certain number of hours. Consider this as a training period.

Do Your Research

Read up as much as you can about intermittent fasting; this way it will put to rest any uncertainties you might have and introduce you to new ways of getting through a fasting day. Check out recipes that won't make you feel like a rabbit having to chomp on carrots all day if you are stuck with ideas of what to eat.

Have Fun

Lastly, have fun, and see what your body can do, even over 50. It is important to know that just because you are a certain age doesn't mean you are incapable of pursuing a new lifestyle change. Reward yourself when it is due, track your progress, adjust where need be, and **get your beauty sleep**. This is another secret to achieving overall wellness and happiness.

Know Your BMI

Your **BMI is based on the measurements of your weight and height**; thus, you can easily determine your body mass index, or BMI as it is more commonly known.

In total, there are four categories that an individual can fall into based on this figure. That is underweight, healthy, overweight, and obese. The concept is simple: our BMI gives us quantifiable amounts when comparing our height with our fat, muscles, bones, and organs.

How to Calculate Your BMI

To calculate your BMI, equate your weight (lbs) x 703 divided by your height (in).

Once you have determined your BMI, you can compare it to the body mass index chart to determine which category you are classed into [32].

Class	Your BMI Score
Underweight	less than 18.5 points
Normal weight	18.5 - 24.9 points
Overweight	25 - 29.9 points
Class 1 - Obesity	30 - 34.9 points
Class 2 - Obesity	35 - 39.9 points
Class 3 - Extreme obesity	40+ points

If you find yourself in a category that displeases you, **fasting can help you lower your BMI** and track your progress with the use of the index.

What Is the Glycemic Index?

The glycemic index (GI) is the rank given to foods, specifically carbohydrates, and how it affects your body's blood sugar levels. Not all carbs are the same and can either spike your sugar levels or keep them steady throughout the day. This is based on what and when you are eating.

Carbohydrates that have been ranked below 55 on the Index allow your body to digest them far more slowly, meaning your blood sugar stays moderated and is less likely to cause an increase in your insulin. The opposite is true for carbs on the higher end of the Index.

All foods can be grouped into three categories; they are:

- **Green:** Food with a GI count of 55 and less.
- **Orange:** Food with a GI count of between 59 and 69.
- **Red:** Food with a GI count of 70 and over.

There is a complete list of glycemic food lists online and you are encouraged to make yourself familiar with them. For the benefit of your health, it would be wise to stay within the green category as these foods are low GI, as well as nutrient and vitamin rich. The items found on the red list are best to be avoided as far as possible.

Following a low GI way of eating can help with weight loss, help manage weight, and prevent and manage diabetes.

People with diseases such as heart disease and inflammatory diseases, such as lupus, can also benefit from eating low GI foods.

Further benefits include:

- Sustained energy levels.
- A boost in your brain's mental performance.
- Staves of your risk from developing breast cancer.
- Low GI may prevent age-related eyesight problems.

How to Go Low GI

Drink plenty of water: Stay hydrated and drink plenty of water throughout the day. Say no to sodas or drinks that contain added sugars in them. If you are going to have a glass of alcohol, stick to one or two glasses a day.

Swap out your potatoes: You won't have to avoid white potatoes but make a wise choice and purchase GiLICIOUS potatoes instead. These potatoes have a lower GI ranking.

Alternatively, if you are looking to make mash potatoes, consider halving the mixture with mashed cannellini beans instead.

Dairy: Dairy is good for your health as it is rich in calcium. Levels of calcium in women begin to drop as they age, so it is important to drink and eat foods rich in this vitamin. Opt for low or non-fat dairy options and avoid rice milks, which have a high GI count.

Grains: Stay away from your baked goods that use white flour. If you can see the grains and seeds in the bread or baked goods, the better.

Rice: Rice such as jasmine has a high GI count. If you are going to eat rice, choose to cook basmati instead, or half the rice portion with a portion of brown rice instead.

Breakfast cereals: Get rid of processed breakfast cereals in your house. Stick to eating muesli, granola, oats, and porridge.

Snack time: Eat fresh fruits with their peels and all on if you can when looking to snack on something. Dried fruit is ok too, but avoid those that have been laced with sugar or sweeteners.

Be smart: Vinegar is known to lower the GI levels of foods; drizzle some over your salad. Opt to eat yogurt with your fruits and consider adding lemon juice to your vegetables.

Legume love: Eat legumes two to three times a week, and if you are a vegan or vegetarian, this amount should be increased. They are a universal food and can be used to make pâtés and spreads, and it can be added to stews and baked meals. They are high in protein and fiber, which are important elements of any meal.

Fasting Q and A

If I fast, does that mean I can't drink anything in between?

No, you make continue to keep up your fluids throughout the day. Stick to water or black tea or coffee.

Will fasting hamper my metabolism?

No, it does the opposite; it fuels your metabolism and allows your body to tap in stored fat reserves.

I know I will lose weight but what about the loss of muscle mass?

Any diet will help you lose weight but will also affect your muscle mass. The best recommendation is to strength train once or twice a week and eat plenty of lean protein. Intermittent fasting has been known to cause less muscle loss than other, traditional forms of dieting.

Should I stop taking my supplements?

No, continue as you were before, though do take them with meals.

Can I use sweeteners?

Yes, but remember that they are not real foods.

How to Plan Round-Up

- Use a calendar.
- Make use of a journal.
- Plan your meals and cook your fasting meals a day before the time.
- Know your measurements.
- Congratulate yourself on the small successes.

- Learn to say "no" to the food you do not need.
- Learn to know when you are full.
- Start exercising.
- Track and trace your BMI.
- Make use of apps.
- Practice mindful eating and portion control.

Are you enjoying this book? If so, I'd be really happy if you could leave a short review on Amazon. It means a lot to me! Thank you.

Chapter 5: Fasting Food Lists

"Your body is your temple, keep it pure and clean for the soul to reside in." - B.K.S. Iyengar

The 21st century with all of its modern-day conveniences are also slowing down our weight loss and impacting how long we live.

Many might ask, how can fasting become part of my lifestyle if I have to cut almost everything I enjoy out of it such as alcohol, chocolate, sugar, and fats? What will be left for me to savor if all the "nice" stuff is to be avoided? The answer is everything in moderation and to stay within the 500 calorie mark on the days that you fast, **eat foods that are low GI, and high levels of lean protein**. The reason for this is because these foods make you feel fuller for longer, leaving you less inclined to tuck into a chocolate bar.

Because you go between days of fasting and not, the regimen is easy to implement into your pre-existing one. Once you begin (and over time), it will become easier and your body will adapt to the fasting cycle.

Your Shopping List

Items on your shopping list should include the following; they are all low on the glycemic index and carry lesser amounts of sugar.

Beverages	Dairy	Meats and Seafood		Vegetables	
Black coffee	1% milk	Canned salmon	Minced beef	Asparagus	Cucumber
Black tea	Almond milk	Canned tuna	Minced pork	Beetroot	Eggplant
Cappuccino with skimmed milk	Fruit yogurt	Chicken liver	Mussels	Bell peppers Bok choy	Kale Leek
Diet coke	Low-fat cottage cheese	Cod	Pre-packed sliced ham	Broccoli	Lettuce (all)
Latte with skimmed milk	Low-fat creme fraiche	Egg	Skinless duck breast	Cabbage	Mushrooms
Lime juice	Low-fat yogurt	Fresh tuna	Skinless chicken breast	Carrot	Red/white onion
Low-calorie hot chocolate	Skim milk	Lean beef	Skinless turkey	Cauliflower	Spinach
Orange squash	Soy milk	Lean ham	Sole	Celery	Tomato
Water	Whole milk	Lean pork	Stewing beef	Chard	Zucchini

Fruit		Sauces, toppings, and dressings	Nuts	Grains and Cereals
Apple	Orange	Basil and tomato sauce	All	Brown rice
Banana	Papaya	Capers	**Seeds**	Bulgur wheat
Blackberries	Peach	Gherkins	All	Couscous
Blueberries	Pear	Jalapeños	**Pulses**	Oats
Cherries	Pineapple	Low-calorie salad dressing	All	Polenta
Cranberries	Plum	Low-fat mayonnaise	**Herbs and spices**	Quinoa
Grapefruit	Raspberries	Olives	All	
Grapes	Strawberries	Pickles	**Fats**	
Kiwi	Tangerine	Pickled onions	Avocado oil	
Lemon	Watermelon	Ready-made gravy	Extra-virgin olive oil	
Lime		Red and white vinegar	Grape seed oil	
Melon		Salsa	Sesame seed oil	

Enjoy the Following Foods

Coffee

You won't have to cut the coffee, just skip the lattes and cappuccinos. Coffee is not bad for you; it is how we drink it that affects the body. Choose to drink it with sweetener and low-fat milk rather than with full cream milk and sugar. Coffee is one of the few things people are willing to give up.

Caffeine, the compound found in coffee, is actually why we love the drink so much; it is responsible for numbing the receptors of the brain that make us drowsy, thus making us feel energized. After 15 minutes of drinking a cup, it will begin to work on the brain.

Coffee is also a diuretic (causing the increase of urine production) and is known to impact the digestive system.

Chocolate

Chocolate is not bad for us either, just the choice in chocolate and our will-power that is bad for us. **Stay away from white chocolate; it is not real chocolate** and opt for darker variants, like 70% cocoa and above. A tad of indulgence is good for you; it boosts your mood too, so have a nibble, but not the whole slab.

Alcohol

Calorie-friendly options include red wine, champagne, gin, and whiskey. Alcohol has the opposite effect on our bodies than caffeine and that is because it tampers with our levels of concentration. Whereas coffee peps us up, one drink can wind us down. These effects happen 30 minutes after consuming a glass of bubbles or a drink of choice.

If you are going to have a glass or shot on your fast day, make sure it complies with your calorie count for the day. However, it is best avoided on fasting days.

Nuts

Nuts are satisfying and can help keep the hunger pangs away on the days that you fast. Stick with options such as cashews, almonds, and pistachios. Remember, go easy on the nuts; they are healthy for you but too many can impact your calorie count on fast days. A small handful will do and should help you feel more comfortable if you happen to be struggling with hunger pains.

Seeds

Nibble on larger seeds like a handful of pumpkin seeds or sprinkle raw seeds over salads and roasted vegetables. Sesame and sunflower seeds are popular and are loaded with important vitamins such as zinc, iron, and good fats.

Grains and Cereals

Stick with oats, couscous, brown rice, quinoa, polenta, or bulgur wheat. These foods are low in GI and high in fiber, aiding your digestion and helping you to stay regular. These are important factors when eating healthy and moderating your energy levels.

Herbs and Spices

All are on the green list, so include them wherever you can. They improve the taste of your food. Dishes can be altered by adding a variety of spices and herbs, which may prevent you from getting bored at mealtimes.

Vegetables

Leafy greens such as kale and spinach are your top choices when it comes to your vegetable options, as well as all variants of lettuce too. Green beans are just as healthy for you and are rich in omega-three fatty acids.

Fruit

Stick with your citrus fruits such as lemons, limes, oranges, grapefruit, and tangerines. Certain minerals found in citrus fruits such as grapefruit support the liver by burning fat rather than holding onto it. Be warned though that grapefruit, in particular, can cause contraindications with medications, so check in with your local doctor, especially if you are taking statins. If this does not sound like something you would like to risk, then opt for an apple or a slice of watermelon.

Tomatoes also contain high levels of minerals and nutrients that protect the body from cancers. Munch on an assortment of berries, which are high in antioxidants and rich in vitamin C. Eat all fruits, skin, core, and pips where you can.

Water

Water is necessary for your overall health. Humans lose plenty of it during the day and to maintain an equilibrium, we need to replenish what was lost.

Water does many things; it lends a hand in digestion, allows the nutrients within our bodies to be transported to where they need to be, and aids circulation. All of these things begin to slow down with age.

Most importantly, water affects our skin; being dehydrated causes our skin to become discolored and dry, and are things we wish to avoid as we age.

Foods to Avoid

Added sugar

Skip the fizzy drinks; there are on average eight teaspoons of sugar found in one can of soda. That is a lot when you add up your sugar intake over the whole day. The rule of thumb is to only take in six teaspoons of sugar or less than one ounce over the whole period of the day and even less if you can. This total is made up of the sugar we add to food and the sugar already found in foods.

It is also best to stay away from sweeteners. Sugar occurs in all the food we eat: processed, unprocessed, and naturally occurring like that in milk, honey, fruits, and vegetables.

Did you know the human brain burns sugar? It needs it to function, so it is still a very fundamental part of our livelihood. The "bad" sugars that are usually brought up in diet conversations are those found in sugars and syrups added to processed foods.

When we eat fruits, vegetables, and other natural foods with sugar, we are getting not just the sweetness from them but also all their other, good, whole-some nutrients. When we eat processed foods or add sugar to our cereals and drinks, we are consuming empty calories, which do nothing good for our bodies.

Fats

Regarded as the worst thing we could consume and tremendously bad for our health and waistlines. **Fats found in food contribute twice as many calories than sugars and proteins.** The misconception is that eating "fatty" foods means we are wider and heavier than most, the same as eating a low-fat diet contributing to weight-loss. Obviously, if we combine a low-fat with a restricted calorie intake, weight-loss will occur.

Consuming more than what our body needs will make anybody gain weight, regardless of what we eat. If we consume more than what is needed, our body hoards this fat as a fail-safe, so when hunger strikes, we aren't satiated and the body will then feed off this fat storage. A healthy metabolism is there to burn this fat, and less calorie intake means our bodies begin to naturally consume the fat sitting neatly above the waistband of our jeans. Read the packaging and avoid anything with trans-fats at all costs.

Processed Foods

Processed foods are considered a threat to your health, and it is one of the main factors that contribute to illness and obesity.

In general, the majority of the food we eat is processed in some way, shape, or form. For example, butter is created from cream, fruits are plucked from the branches, and meats are minced. There is, however, a stark difference between what has been chemically processed versus mechanically processed.

Consider this rule of thumb: if the item is the sole ingredient found in the jar, without any other chemicals and sugars added, then it is still considered the real deal when it comes to food.

Processed foods are full of empty calories and high in sugars. They are also modified with chemicals to stabilize them and prepare them for the market. These chemicals are also there to ensure longer shelf life too. Flavors are added but not the real thing, making it artificial. These foods also have little to no fiber in them, nor any other benefits.

What makes the whole situation worse is that you can become addicted to processed foods.

Herbal Teas for Better Health

Intermittent fasting can be tough on certain days and keeping up your fluids is one way to help your body while fasting, and it is also important to consume fluids on your regular, non-fasting days.

Staying hydrated can be difficult if you are not someone who drinks a lot of water or prefers to drink tea and coffee with milk and sugar but have chosen to avoid these beverages while fasting because you cannot stomach black tea and coffee.

Herbal teas could be an alternative option when it comes to keeping up your fluids. Apart from that, they are easy to drink, can be enjoyed hot or cold, and benefit our health.

Before exploring the aisles and wide range of herbal teas available, it is best to read the package before purchasing. Do not buy any teas with added colorants, sugars, and flavors. Herbal tea should just be that, herbal.

As herbs go, they have been considered medicinal for centuries and can be self-prescribed to treat certain ailments.

For Balancing Hormones

White peony: Is considered an estrogen modulator and can ease any fluid retention or bloating that you might have.

Spearmint: Eases stomach upsets, cramps, and nausea. Drink spearmint three times a day. Purchase fresh spearmint, tear off a few leaves, place them into a cup and pour boiling water over them; enjoying it as simply as this!

For Your Liver

Nettle leaf: Nettle is rich in silica, iron, and potassium and it is used for treating inflammation.

St. Mary's thistle: Thistle tea is known to restore the cells within the liver and protect it. It is also a novel herbal tea for treating headaches.

Dandelion root: Dandelion root stimulates your digestive system and cleans the body of any excess hormonal build-up, which may cause mood swings and low energy levels.

For Stress Management

Licorice: Exhausted, moody, and/or have hot flushes? Drink a cup of hot licorice tea to ease these symptoms.

Chamomile: Reduce inflammation and restore calm. Chamomile may ease your stress and welcome a restful night's sleep.

Aids Digestion

Cinnamon: Regulate your blood sugar levels with a cup of cinnamon tea.

Fennel seed: For those who struggle with IBS (irritable bowel syndrome), fennel seed tea has been known to help ease the symptoms and help relieve those who find themselves fatigued.

Lemon: Lemon tea is great for fueling your metabolism as it supports weight-loss, and it is wonderful for supporting liver and kidney function too. Lemon is also high in vitamin C, so drinking a cup will help fight infections.

Supplements to Support Your Health After 50

Supplements are there to support your health and are not the answer to curing illness or sickness. If you are concerned about any of the effects they might cause, be sure to contact your doctor or health-care practitioner for advice.

Some supplements might prove beneficial in terms of aging, such as calcium that can stave off osteoporosis in women.

It is important to know that a supplement is either one or more combinations of amino acids, vitamins, minerals, herbs, and botanicals combined to prevent and support aging, nutritional shortages, health, and overall well-being.

Below are suggested supplements to consider taking along with the foods that are most rich in the mentioned nutrient.

Probiotics: The impact the gut can have on your health is plentiful; therefore, it makes sense to protect it and keep it functioning in a balanced manner. There is nothing worse than battling with IBS or diarrhea. Probiotics safeguards against these. Probiotics naturally occur on yogurt, so ensure your diet does consist of a few helpings each or every other day.

Omega-3: Omega-3 is a rich, fatty acid that can stave off developing heart disease and may even help you avoid developing rheumatoid arthritis. Omega-3 is naturally found in fish such as salmon and trout. Consider incorporating fish into your weekly eating regime at least two to three times a week.

Calcium: Calcium naturally occurs in our bones but gradually begins to decline as we age. Women can especially become prone to developing osteoporosis if these levels are low or dwindling. Milk and yogurt are rich sources of calcium, so are leafy greens, especially spinach and kale, and legumes and almonds.

Vitamin B12: Keep your blood cells and nerve cells healthy by getting enough vitamin B12. Food rich in this vitamin are lean proteins and fish. Aging can determine how quickly you absorb and utilize B12. Apart from seeking it in food, it would be wise to consider taking a B12 supplement to assist in absorbing the amount your body needs, in particular, if you are over the age of 50.

Vitamin D: Sunshine, you are my only sunshine. This wonder vitamin helps you absorb calcium and phosphorus. A vitamin D supplement taken after the age of 50 might help prevent loss in bone mass and prevent bone breaks. Getting a few rays uplifts your mood, so it would be wise sitting in the sun for a few minutes a day; ensure you wear your hat and sunscreen. Alternatively, take a 20 to 30 minutes' walk each day to improve your vitamin D levels.

Vitamin C: Helps heal wounds, prevents cataracts from developing, and can up your immune system. Seek vitamin C in all citrus, and broccoli and bell peppers are rich in this vitamin, so make sure your diet includes lots of this fresh produce.

Magnesium: Keep teeth and bones healthy by adding magnesium to your diet. Magnesium is needed by the body so it can unlock calcium, which is then sent to the bones to do its work. Magnesium is also said to aid with energy levels and helps detoxify the body. It has also been suggested it can help those who suffer from sleeplessness, anxiety, and migraines.

Magnesium does not need to be taken in supplement form but an individual can bathe in a magnesium salt bath; the skin readily absorbs this. Trying taking a salt bath after exercising as it aids in the body's ability to recover and restore itself after physical activity. Coffee, alcohol, and sugar can cause the body to get rid of magnesium reserves through urine, so it is wise to limit the intake of these items. Asparagus, green beans, peas, and broccoli are rich with magnesium, so be sure to include them into your diet often.

Fasting Food Round-Up

- Avoid processed foods.
- Say no to sugar.
- Eat lean meat.
- Stick with the low- or non-fat options.
- Drink plenty of water.
- Opt for low GI food options.
- Count your calories.

- Drink herbal teas to stay hydrated.

- Buy fresh, wholesome ingredients, fruits, and vegetables.

- Stockpile your pantry and refrigerator with fresh herbs and spices.

Chapter 6: Recipes to Enjoy

"Good food is very often, even most often, simple food." - Anthony Bourdain

A ll these recipes below are fasting-friendly and combine a range of fresh, wholesome ingredients that are affordable and easily located at your nearest supermarket.

Alter the recipes to suit your tastes and calorie intake. All the recipes mentioned are under 500 calories, well under the restricted fasting day requirements.

Get creative with ingredients and remember to enjoy yourself in the kitchen; your food will show this and eating it will be far more satisfying than a few measly stalks of celery and chopped carrots on a plate.

Smoothies

Summer Watermelon Smoothie

Preparation time: 5 minutes

Total cook time: 5 minutes

Serving size: 2 servings

Ingredients:

- ½ cup of ice cubes
- ½ cup of low-fat milk
- 1 teaspoon of lemon juice
- 1 cup of strawberries
- 1 ½ cups of watermelon
- Sweetener of your choice to taste

Directions:

1. Add all of the ingredients into a blender. Pulse until combined and there are no lumps. Enjoy served in a tall glass.

Calories: 95 kcal per serving.

Tip(s):

1. As an alternative, use half a cup of strawberries and half a cup of blueberries.

Tropical Smoothie

Preparation time: 5 minutes

Total cook time: 5 minutes

Serving size: 2 servings

Ingredients:

- ½ cup of almond milk, unsweetened
- ½ a banana
- ½ cup of mango
- ½ cup of spinach
- ½ cup of kale

Directions:

1. In a blender, add in all the ingredients. Pulse until smooth and serve

Calories: 70 kcal per serving.

Tip(s):

1. For those hot summer days, add a cup of ice cubes to your blender along with the rest of the ingredients.

Green Smoothie

Preparation time: 5 minutes

Total cook time: 5 minutes

Serving size: 2 servings

Ingredients:

- 1 cup of almond milk, unsweetened
- 1 tablespoon of ground flaxseeds
- 1 cup of pear
- 2 cups of spinach leaves

Directions:

1. Place all of the ingredients into a blender. Blend until smooth, and then serve.

Calories: 85 kcal per serving.

Tip(s):

1. As an alternative, consider using one cup of spinach leaves and one cup of kale leaves instead.

Rise and Shine Smoothie

Preparation time: 5 minutes

Total cook time: 5 minutes

Serving size: 2 servings

Ingredients:

- 2 bananas
- 2 ½ cups of fresh orange juice
- 1 cup of low- or non-fat yogurt
- 2 ½ cups of frozen berries

Directions:

1. Once the ingredients are placed into a blender, pulse until smooth, and then serve.

Calories: 139 kcal per serving.

Tip(s):

1. Add sweetener to taste.

Lemon and Blueberry Smoothie

Preparation time: 5 minutes

Total cook time: 5 minutes

Serving size: 2 servings

Ingredients:

- 1 ½ cups of chilled water
- ⅔ cups of coconut milk
- ½ cup of fresh lemon juice
- 2 cups of frozen blueberries

Directions:

1. In a blender, add the ingredients. Pulse until the mixture is smooth, pour into two tall drinking glasses, and serve.

Calories: 100 kcal per serving.

Tip(s):

1. Choose to buy fresh coconut milk as the canned variety contains more calories.

Carrot and Orange Smoothie

Preparation time: 5 minutes

Total cook time: 5 minutes

Serving size: 2 servings

Ingredients:

- 2 cups of ice-cubes
- 1 ½ cups of orange juice
- ½ cup of diced carrots
- 2 teaspoons of minced ginger

Directions:

1. Once the ingredients are in a blender., pulse everything until combined, and then serve.

Calories: 97 kcal per serving.

Tip(s):

1. Add a few drops of honey to sweeten the smoothie.

Breakfast

Tomato, Spinach, and Baked Eggs

Preparation time: 10 minutes

Total cook time: 20 minutes

Serving size: 4 servings

Ingredients:

- 1 pinch of salt
- 1 pinch of ground, black pepper
- 1 teaspoon of dried, chili flakes
- 4 eggs
- 1 can of diced tomatoes
- 3.5 oz. of fresh spinach

Directions:

1. **Preheat your oven to 350 °F Grease 4 oven-proof dishes with extra-virgin olive oil.**
2. Rinse off the spinach and place it into a colander. Pour boiling water over the spinach to wilt them.
3. Drain the spinach and divide equally between the 4 dishes.
4. In a separate dish, combine the salt, pepper, chili flakes, and canned tomato. Evenly dish the tomato over the spinach.
5. Crack an egg over each dish and bake in the oven for about 15 minutes or until the eggs have reached the consistency you prefer.

Calories: 114 kcal per serving.

Tip(s):

1. Add in finely diced shallots and garlic to add flavor.

Blueberry Breakfast Porridge

Preparation time: 10 minutes

Total cook time: 10 minutes

Serving size: 2 servings

Ingredients:

- Agave to taste
- 13.5 fl. oz. of water
- 3.3 fl. oz. of low-fat Greek style yogurt
- 12 oz. of frozen blueberries
- 6 tablespoons of oats

Directions:

1. In a frying pan, over medium heat, add in the water and oats. Cook for two minutes or until cooked. Remove from heat and add in half of the yogurt.
2. In a separate, small saucepan, add the blueberries and allow them to thaw. Add in any sweetener if desired.
3. To serve, dish the oats up into servings bowls, top with the heated blueberries and the remainder of the yogurt.

Calories: 168 kcal per serving.

Tip(s):

1. Halve the frozen blueberries with an equal portion of frozen strawberries or raspberries.

Spinach, Tomato, and Ricotta Frittata

Preparation time: 15 minutes

Total cook time: 25 minutes

Serving size: 4 servings

Ingredients:

- 1 pinch of salt
- 1 pinch of ground, black pepper
- 1 tablespoon of extra-virgin olive oil
- 6 eggs
- 3.5 oz. ricotta
- 1 onion, finely diced
- 3.5 oz. of spinach leaves
- 10.5 oz. of cherry tomatoes
- A handful of fresh basil leaves

Directions:

1. **Preheat your oven to 350 °F Grease a 9" x 13" baking tin.**
2. Over medium heat, in a large frying pan, add the oil and onion. Cook for five minutes or until tender. Add the tomatoes and let them cook for a further minute.
3. Remove the pan from the heat, add in the salt, pepper, and spinach leaves. Allow the leaves to wilt by stirring them in gently with the rest of the mixture.
4. Add the mixture to the baking tin, then top the vegetables with the ricotta.
5. Beat the eggs and then pour over the vegetables. Bake in the oven for 25 minutes or until cooked.

Calories: 236 kcal per serving.

Tip(s):

1. Add ½ teaspoon of finely diced garlic when frying off the onion.

Soft Boiled Egg With Asparagus-Styled Soldiers

Preparation time: 15 minutes

Total cook time: 15 minutes

Serving size: 4 servings

Ingredients:

- 1 pinch of salt
- 1 pinch of black, ground pepper
- 1 pinch of chili
- 1 pinch of paprika
- 1 tablespoon of extra-virgin olive oil
- 4 large eggs
- 30 spears of asparagus
- 2 oz. of dried breadcrumbs

Directions:

1. In a frying pan that is medium in size, over medium heat, add the olive oil and breadcrumbs. Fry until golden and crispy, and then add the salt, pepper, chili, and paprika; combine well then set aside.
2. In a medium saucepan, over medium heat, cover the asparagus with water and boil until tender; then remove from the water and set aside.
3. In a separate saucepan, boil the eggs for 4 minutes.
4. To dish up, stand 1 egg in a holder onto each plate, evenly divide the asparagus, and then sprinkle with the breadcrumbs.

Calories: 186 kcal per serving.

Tip(s):

1. Asparagus is rich in folic acid and a good antioxidant to include on the days that you both fast and eat regularly.

Egg White Omelet

Preparation time: 5 minutes

Total cook time: 5 minutes

Serving size: 1 serving

Ingredients:

- 1 pinch of salt
- 1 pinch of black, ground pepper
- 1 teaspoon of extra-virgin olive oil
- 3 egg whites
- 2 teaspoons of milk

Directions:

1. In a mixing bowl, separate the egg yolks from the egg whites.
2. Add the salt, pepper, and milk to the egg white and whisk, using a hand whisk until light and frothy.
3. In a small frying pan, add the olive oil and egg white.
4. Allow to cook until it sets; add a filling of your choice.
5. Using a spatula, flip one half of the omelet over the ingredients and then slide onto a plate, and serve.

Calories: Under 100 kcal per serving.

Tip(s):

1.   Skip the dairy and add 2 teaspoons of water to the recipe instead.
2.   Add ham, chicken, or diced onion and tomato as filling options. Fresh herbs also go a long way to lifting the flavors of the dish without adding extra calories.

Stuffed Avocados

Preparation time: 15 minutes

Total cook time: 35 minutes

Serving size: 4 servings

Ingredients:

- 1 pinch of salt
- 1 pinch of black, ground pepper
- 2 avocados, halved and pitted
- 3 slices of bacon
- 4 eggs
- ⅓cup of fresh chives

Directions:

1.   Preheat your oven to 350 °F
2.   Place the halved avocados onto a baking tray, facing upwards.
3.   Crack the eggs open into a bowl; do this gently to prevent the egg yolk from seeping.
4.   Scoop one yolk into each hole where the avocado pip was. Drizzle the egg white over the yolk as much as the space can accommodate.
5.   Place into the oven. Bake until the whites have set. Remove from the oven and set aside.

6. In a small frying pan, fry off the bacon until crispy; remove from heat and place bacon onto a kitchen towel to soak up any excess fats. Dice and sprinkle evenly over the four filled avocado halves.

7. Season with salt, pepper, and a sprinkle of fresh chives.

Calories: 220 kcal per serving.

Tip(s):

1. If your avocado begins to brown in the oven, cover them with tinfoil to prevent them from discoloring.

Lunch

Thai Inspired Pineapple and Chicken Salad

Preparation time: 10 minutes

Total cook time: 15 minutes

Serving size: 2 servings

Ingredients:

- 1 pinch of salt
- 1 pinch of ground, black pepper
- 2 tablespoons of white wine vinegar
- 1 tablespoon of chili sauce
- 5 oz. of cooked chicken breast, store-bought, flavors include bbq and lemon and herb
- 8 oz. of canned pineapple, finely diced
- 1 red onion, finely diced
- 1 chili, deseeded and finely sliced
- 3 oz. of mixed lettuce leaves
- 1 cup of cherry tomatoes

- A handful of fresh cilantro

Directions:

1. Drain the canned pineapple and retain the juice.
2. In a large salad bowl, combine slithers of cooked chicken, diced pineapple, onion, lettuce, cherry tomatoes, and cilantro.
3. In a separate bowl, combine the salt, pepper, vinegar, chili sauce, diced chili, and 2 tablespoons of the retained pineapple juice. Whisk together.
4. Drizzle the sauce over the salad and serve.

Calories: 176 kcal per serving.

Tip(s):

1. Add a handful of raw, mixed nuts for added texture.

Moroccan Soup

Preparation time: 10 minutes

Total cook time: 25 minutes

Serving size: 4 servings

Ingredients:

- 1 pinch of salt
- 1 pinch of ground, black pepper
- 2 teaspoons of ground cumin
- 20 fl. oz. of vegetable stock
- 1 tablespoon of extra-virgin olive oil
- 1 clove of garlic, finely diced
- 1 onion, finely diced
- 2 stalks of celery, diced
- 1 can of chickpeas, drained and rinsed

- 1 can of plum tomatoes
- 3.5 oz. of frozen broad-beans
- Zest and juice of ½ a lemon
- A handful of fresh cilantro

Directions:

1. Over medium heat, in a large saucepan, add the onion, celery, garlic, salt, pepper, and oil. Cook for five minutes or until the onion softens. Add in the cumin and cook for another minute.
2. Increase the heat to high, add the stock, chickpeas, and canned tomatoes. Turn the heat down to a simmer. Cook for a further 10 minutes.
3. Add in the lemon juice and beans; cook for two minutes.
4. To serve, top with the lemon zest and fresh cilantro.

Calories: 150 kcal per serving.

Tips:

1. Add shredded, cooked chicken breast to turn this into a hearty wintertime meal.

Mixed Vegetable and Feta Tart

Preparation time: 15 minutes

Total cook time: 45 minutes

Serving size: 4 servings

Ingredients:

- 1 pinch of salt
- 1 pinch of ground, black pepper
- 1 teaspoon of dried oregano

- 2 tablespoons of extra-virgin olive oil
- 3 tablespoons of balsamic vinegar
- 2 zucchinis, sliced
- 1 eggplant, sliced
- 2 red onions, sliced
- ¾ cup of cherry tomatoes, halved
- 3 sheets of phyllo pastry
- 3.5 oz. of feta cheese

Directions:

1. **Preheat your oven to 400 °F and place a 13" by 9" baking tin into the oven to heat up.**
2. In a griddle pan, over medium heat, add the oil. Grill the eggplant and zucchini slices, until evenly charred. Continue to do the same with the slices of onion. Set this all aside once cooked.
3. Remove the heated tray from the oven and grease with olive oil. Brush one sheet of phyllo pastry with oil, place it into the pan and repeat until all have been brushed and layered upon one another in the baking tin.
4. Layer the charred vegetables, add a pinch of salt and pepper, and then sprinkle the cherry tomatoes evenly over the charred vegetables. Drizzle with the balsamic vinegar, crumble the feta over, and finely add a dash of the oregano.
5. Bake for 25 minutes or until the pastry turns a golden color, then serve!

Calories: 195 kcal per serving.

Tip(s):

1. Serve with a fresh salad of mixed lettuce leaves and a coating of balsamic vinegar to round off the meal.

Sweet Potato and Red Lentil Pâté

Preparation time: 15 minutes

Total cook time: 35 minutes

Serving size: 4 servings

Ingredients:

- 1 pinch of salt
- 1 pinch of black, ground pepper
- 1 teaspoon of paprika
- 1 tablespoon of extra-virgin olive oil
- 1 teaspoon of red wine vinegar
- 17 fl. oz. of vegetable stock
- ½ of an onion, finely diced
- 1 sweet potato, peeled and diced
- 5 oz. of red lentil
- 3 sprigs of fresh thyme

Directions:

1. In a large saucepan and over medium heat, add the olive oil and onion. Cook until the onion becomes tender. Add the salt, pepper, and paprika and cook for a further 2 minutes. Add the lentils, sweet potato, fresh thyme, and stock.
2. Bring the mixture to a boil and then allow to simmer until the vegetables are cooked through, so about 20 minutes.
3. Add the red wine vinegar and then mash the mixture until smooth. Set in the refrigerator for 1 hour, remove, and add 1 teaspoon of extra-virgin olive oil. Serve with sliced celery and carrot sticks.

Calories: 200 kcal per serving.

Tip(s):

1. Sprinkle the prepared pâté with more paprika and fresh herbs for added flavor.

Roasted Cauliflower

Preparation time: 15 minutes

Total cook time: 1 hour

Serving size: 4 servings

Ingredients:

- 1 pinch of salt
- 1 pinch of black, ground pepper
- 1 pinch of paprika
- 1 pinch of chili powder
- 1 pinch of cinnamon
- 1 pinch of ras el hanout
- 3.3 fl. oz. of water
- Juice of 2 lemons
- 1 teaspoon of extra-virgin olive oil
- 2 tablespoons of tahini
- 6 oz. of low- or non-fat Greek yogurt
- 1 clove of garlic, finely diced
- 1 cauliflower, rinsed off
- 14 oz. of canned chickpeas, rinsed and drained

Directions:

1. Preheat your oven to 350 °F and grease a baking tin.
2. In a mixing bowl, combine the salt, pepper, spices, oil, and yogurt.
3. Place the cauliflower, minus leaves and stalk, into the baking tin. Gently rub the yogurt mixture all over the cauliflower.

4. Pour the water around the cauliflower and then cover with tinfoil. Place into the oven and bake for 45 minutes.

5. In a separate bowl, combine the tahini and lemon juice. Using a hand whisk, blend until it reaches a smooth consistency. Set this aside in the refrigerator.

6. After the cook time has come to an end for the cauliflower, remove it from the oven, remove the tinfoil, and set the cauliflower back into the oven for a further 10 minutes.

7. In a medium saucepan, add the chickpeas, add one tablespoon of water, and cook on high until the chickpeas are hot to the touch. Remove from the heat. Add one pinch of salt and pepper and using a masher, mash until smooth. Add one teaspoon of the rested tahini sauce and give it a good stir.

8. Cut the cauliflower into eight pieces.

9. Top one oven-warmed, whole-wheat pita bread with mashed chickpea, followed by a piece of the cauliflower and drizzled with the tahini sauce.

Calories: 194 kcal per serving.

Tip(s):

1. Mexican taco spice will also work in place of ras el hanout.

2. Serve the meal with pumpkin seeds, fresh mint, flat-leaf parsley, and fresh pomegranate seeds.

Tomato Soup

Preparation time: 35 minutes

Total cook time: 50 minutes

Serving size: 6 servings

Ingredients:

- 1 pinch of salt
- 1 pinch of black, ground pepper
- 1 pinch of paprika
- 4 bay leaves
- 3 vegetable stock cubes
- 2 tablespoons of brown sugar
- 3 tablespoons of extra-virgin olive oil
- 5 tablespoons of tomato puree
- 2 tablespoons of red wine vinegar
- 13.5 fl. oz. of low-fat milk
- 17 oz. of potato, peeled and diced; choose "*GiLICIOUS*" potatoes if available
- 11 oz. of carrots, peeled and diced
- 2 sticks of celery, diced
- 2 onions, diced
- 4 x 4 canned diced tomato
- 17 oz. of passata

Directions:

1. In a large casserole dish, over medium heat, add the olive oil, carrots, celery, onion, potato and bay leaves. Fry until the onions become tender. Meanwhile, fill your kettle to the brim with water and boil the water.
2. Add in the passata, tomato puree, red wine vinegar, canned tomato, and sugar. Add in the stock cubes by crumbling them into the mixture. Stir well so all the ingredients are combined.
3. Add 33 fl. oz. of boiling water to this mixture, and salt, pepper, and paprika too. Cover the casserole

and allow the soup to cook until the potato has softened (15 minutes).

4. Remove the bay leaves and using a hand blender, blitz the soup until you reach a smooth consistency. Allow to cool before adding the milk, then reheat and serve.

Calories: 180 kcal per serving.

Tip(s):

1. This soup recipe freezes well; it can be stored in the freezer for three months in an airtight container.

Dinner

Chickpea Curry

Preparation time: 20 minutes

Total cook time: 45 minutes

Serving size: 6 servings

Ingredients:

- 1 pinch of salt
- 1 pinch of ground, black pepper
- 1 pinch of chili flakes
- 1 teaspoon of turmeric
- 1 teaspoon of ground cumin
- 1 teaspoon of yeast extract
- 2 teaspoons of ground coriander
- 1 tablespoon of roasted sesame seeds
- 1 tablespoon of roasted cashews, finely diced
- 1 teaspoon of extra-virgin olive oil
- 6 tablespoons of coconut cream

- 1 knob of ginger, peeled and finely diced
- 2 cloves of garlic, finely diced
- 1 onion, diced
- 6 tomatoes
- Juice of 1 lemon
- 3.5 oz of spinach leaves
- 1 broccoli, broken into florets
- 4 tablespoons of red lentils
- 1 can of chickpeas, rinsed and drained

Directions:

1. Add the ginger, garlic, and tomatoes into a blender. Pulse until a purée forms.
2. Over medium heat, in a large saucepan, add the oil, salt, pepper, and remaining spices. Cook for a minute, stirring occasionally. Add the puree followed by the yeast. Cook for two more minutes.
3. Add in the lentils and coconut cream. Cook until the lentils have softened. Add in the broccoli florets and the remainder of the broccoli.
4. Allow the mixture to cook for five minutes uncovered. Add in the spinach and chickpeas. Add the lemon juice, sesame seeds, and cashew nuts and serve.

Calories: 205 kcal per serving.

Tip(s):

1. For a more aromatic curry feel, free to add in 1 teaspoon of mild curry powder when cooking the other spices in the recipe.

Leafy-Green Soup

Preparation time: 20 minutes

Total cook time: 25 minutes

Serving size: 2 servings

Ingredients:

- 1 pinch of salt
- 1 pinch of ground, black pepper
- ½ teaspoon of turmeric
- ½ teaspoon of ground coriander
- 1 tablespoon of fresh, flat-leaf parsley
- 4 tablespoons of water
- 17 fl. oz. of vegetable stock
- 1 tablespoon of extra-virgin olive oil
- 2 cloves of garlic, diced
- 1 knob of ginger, peeled and finely diced
- 1 lime, juiced and zested
- 3.5 oz. of kale, diced
- 3.5 oz. of broccoli, diced
- 7 oz. of zucchini, diced

Directions:

1. Over medium heat, in a large saucepan, add the oil, salt, pepper, spices, garlic, and ginger. Add the water and combine well.
2. Add the sliced zucchini and cook for five minutes. Follow by adding 13 fl. oz. of stock and allow to simmer for three more minutes, uncovered.
3. Add the lime juice, kale and broccoli, and the remainder of the stock to the saucepan. Cook for five minutes or until the vegetables have become tender.
4. Remove from the heat, add the fresh parsley. Pour the mixture over into a blender, pulse until smooth.
5. Garnish with the zest of the lime and serve.

Calories: 185 kcal per serving.

Tip(s):

1. Alter the recipe by adding half kale and half spinach.

Spicy Bell Pepper Pilafs

Preparation time: 15 minutes

Total cook time: 1 hour

Serving size: 8 servings

Ingredients:

- 1 pinch of salt
- 1 pinch of ground, black pepper
- 1 teaspoon of garam masala
- 1 teaspoon of ground cumin
- 1 knob of fresh ginger, peeled and finely diced
- 2 cloves of garlic, finely diced
- A handful of fresh mint, diced
- 1 tablespoon of extra-virgin olive oil
- 1 teaspoon of tomato puree
- 28 fl. oz. of vegetable stock
- 1 onion, finely diced
- 8 bell peppers
- 7 oz. of spinach leaves, diced
- 5 oz. of red lentils, washed and drained
- 7 oz. basmati rice

Directions:

1. Over medium heat, in a large saucepan, add the oil, salt, pepper, ginger, and garlic; cook until tender.

2. Add the remainder of the spices and the puree and cook for one minute.
3. Add in the rice, combine, and then add the stock, bring to a boil and then allow to simmer. Add in the lentils. Cover the pot with a lid and cook on low heat for 15 minutes or until the lentils have softened.
4. Add in the mint and spinach and set the mixture aside.
5. Preheat your oven to 350 °F and grease a baking tray.
6. Using a sharp knife, remove the tops of the bell peppers, and all white flesh, seeds, and stalks.
7. Fill the bell peppers with the rice mixture and return the "*bell pepper lid.*"
8. For 30 minutes, bake this in the oven or until the peppers have softened.
9. Remove from the oven and serve.

Calories: 210 kcal per serving.

Tip(s):

1. For a tasty extra, add a dollop of low-fat yogurt when serving.

Beetroot and Ham Salad

Preparation time: 20 minutes

Total cook time: 20 minutes

Serving size: 2 servings

Ingredients:

- 1 pinch of salt
- 1 pinch of black, ground pepper
- 2 teaspoons horseradish sauce

- 2 tablespoons of low- or non-fat Greek yogurt
- 3.5 oz. of finely sliced ham
- 6 oz. of beetroot
- 3.5 oz. of frozen peas
- 2 spring onions, finely diced
- Half of an iceberg lettuce, rinsed and shredded

Directions:

1. Dice the cooked or store-bought, prepared beetroot.
2. Place the peas into a bowl and cover with boiling water; allow it to stand like this for 2 minutes.
3. In a separate bowl, add the diced beetroot, spring onions, and drained peas.
4. Combine the horseradish and yogurt; add 1 tablespoon of water to this, give it a good stir, and then drizzle over the salad.
5. Evenly plate the shredded lettuce, top with the salad mixture and ham, then serve.

Calories: 166 kcal per serving.

Tip(s):

1. Use shredded chicken, prawns, tuna, or salmon as a protein alternative.

Stuffed and Baked Marrow

Preparation time: 15 minutes

Total cook time: 1 hour

Serving size: 6 servings

Ingredients:

- 1 pinch of salt
- 1 pinch of black, ground pepper
- 1 tablespoon of dried herbs
- 3 tablespoons of extra-virgin olive oil
- 1 clove of garlic, diced
- 28 oz. of canned diced tomatoes
- 1 onion, finely diced
- 1 large marrow cut into 1.5" slices
- 4 tablespoons of breadcrumbs
- 18 oz. of minced turkey
- 3 tablespoons of shredded Parmesan

Directions:

1. Preheat your oven to 350 °F
2. Over medium heat, in a large saucepan, add the olive oil, onion, garlic, salt, pepper, and two tablespoons of the dried herbs. Cook until the onion becomes tender.
3. Add the minced turkey and fry until browned. Add in the canned tomatoes and continue to cook for a further five minutes.
4. Scoop out the middle of the marrow slices, and discard. Place the marrow slices on a greased baking tin. Then fill the middle of the sliced marrow with the turkey mixture. Cover the marrow with any remaining turkey mixture.
5. Cover with tin foil. Place this in the oven to bake for 30 minutes.
6. In a small mixing bowl, combine the remainder of the herbs, breadcrumbs, and Parmesan cheese.
7. Remove the marrow from the oven once the cooking time comes to an end. Top with the breadcrumb mixture and place back into the oven for a further 10 minutes.

Calories: 198 kcal per serving.

Tip(s):

1. You can also use minced lean beef or pork in place of the minced turkey.

Avocado, Prawn, and Watermelon Salad

Preparation time: 20 minutes

Total cook time: 25 minutes

Serving size: 4 servings

Ingredients:

- 1 pinch of salt
- 1 pinch of black, ground pepper
- 1 red chili, deseeded and finely diced
- 1 clove of garlic, finely diced
- Juice of 1 lime
- 1 tablespoon of rice wine vinegar
- 1 teaspoon of castor sugar
- 1 wedge of watermelon, finely diced
- 1 red onion, finely diced
- 1 avocado, diced
- 7 oz. of cooked tiger prawns
- A handful of fresh cilantro

Directions:

1. In a mixing bowl, combine the lime juice, vinegar, onion, garlic, sugar, salt, and pepper. Stir the mixture and allow it to marinate for 10 to 15 minutes.

2. Combine the remainder of the ingredients in a large serving bowl. Drizzle with the marinade and serve.

Calories: 179 kcal per serving.

Tip(s):

1. Substitute the prawns for shrimp as an alternative.

Dessert

Pineapple Cheesecake Bites

Preparation time: 25 minutes

Total cook time: 4 hours 30 minutes

Serving size: 9 servings

Ingredients for the cheesecake:

- 1 teaspoon of vanilla extract
- ⅓ cup of pineapple juice
- ¾ cup of nonfat Greek yogurt
- 6 oz. of light cream cheese
- 3 eggs
- ¼ cup of white sugar

Ingredients for the crust:

- 2 tablespoons of butter, melted
- ¾ cups of graham crackers, crushed

Directions:

1. Preheat your oven to 300 °F and line a 9" by 9" baking tray with baking parchment. Ensure that the parchment overhangs the edges of the baking tray.

2. In a mixing bowl, combine the crushed crackers and melted butter to form a crust-like mixture.

3. Scoop into the lined baking tray and press flat using a spatula. Place in the oven to bake until golden (5-10 minutes). Once the baking time is up, allow it to cool by removing it from the oven.

4. In a separate mixing bowl, using a hand mixer, beat the cream cheese until smooth. Add in the yogurt and vanilla extract. Beat for a further minute.

5. Add 2 large eggs to the mixture and the yolk of the remaining egg; discard the egg white. Beat on high speed until the mixture is well combined.

6. Add the sugar and pineapple juice.

7. Pour the filling over the pressed crust and place it into the oven. Bake for 30 minutes or until the cheesecake is slightly stiff, and no longer jiggles in the center. Allow it to cool completely in the baking tray after you've removed it from the oven.

8. Place the cooled tray into the refrigerator for 4 hours.

9. To serve, lift the parchment out onto a cutting board. Use a sharp knife to cut 9 squares.

Calories: 130 kcal per serving.

Tip(s):

1. All dairy ingredients should be at room temperature before pursuing this recipe.

2. Store in an airtight container in the refrigerator.

3. Serve with freshly sliced pineapple and cherries for an extra yum factor.

Strawberry Slice

Preparation time: 10 minutes

Total cook time: 4 hours 30 minutes

Serving size: 18 servings

Ingredients for the filling:

- 2 tablespoons of lemon juice
- ¾ cups of brown or white sugar
- 15 0z. of frozen strawberries

Ingredients for the crust:

- ½ cup of coconut sugar
- 1 ½ cups of oat flour
- 6 tablespoons of melted ghee
- ¾ cups of raw pecan nuts, chopped

Directions:

1. Preheat your oven to 375 °F
2. Combine all the ingredients for the crust; scoop this out onto a baking tray. In an oven, bake the crust until golden brown (20 minutes). At the 10-minute mark, remove the tray, stir the crust, and place back into the oven to continue baking.
3. In a separate bowl, using a hand mixer, combine the filling ingredients. Beat on high for 5 to 10 minutes; the mixture should be stiff.
4. In a greased 9" by 13" baking tin, spread the crust mixture evenly using a spatula. Keep one cup of the crust mixture aside.
5. Scoop out the filling mixture and evenly spread it over the crust. Sprinkle the remaining cup of crust mixture over the top, place the baking tin into the refrigerator and allow to set for four hours.

Calories: 130 kcal per serving.

Tip(s):

1. Sprinkle a handful of fresh strawberries over the top when serving.
2. Alter the sugar to your own taste.

Carrot Cake Cups

Preparation time: 15 minutes

Total cook time: 30 minutes

Serving size: 8 large cupcakes

Ingredients:

- 1 pinch of salt
- 1 teaspoon of ground cinnamon
- 1 ½ cups of spelt
- ⅓ cup of unrefined sugar
- 2 tablespoons of brown sugar
- ½ teaspoon of baking soda
- 2 teaspoons of vanilla extract
- 2 teaspoons of apple cider vinegar
- ⅓ cup of extra-virgin olive oil
- ½ cup of applesauce
- 7 oz. of shredded carrot

Directions:

1. Preheat your oven to 350 °F and place 8 cupcake holders into a muffin tray.
2. In a large mixing bowl, combine the dry ingredients.
3. In a separate bowl, add the shredded carrot and stir in the wet ingredients until combined.
4. Combine all of the ingredients (wet with dry) once combined evenly, transfer the mixture into the cupcake holders.

5. Bake for 20 minutes.
6. Remove from the oven, allow to cool in the tray, and then serve.

Calories: 142 kcal per serving.

Tip(s):

1. Add a ½ cup of raisins to the mixture for more flavor.
2. Alternatively, substitute the ⅓cup of oil with ⅓cup of applesauce.
3. Substitute the sugar for stevia, agave, or xylitol. Read the package instructions as you will need to amend how much sweetener you add.

Choc-Chip Blondies

Preparation time: 15 minutes

Total cook time: 35 minutes

Serving size: 12 servings

Ingredients:

- 1 pinch of salt
- 1 pinch of stevia
- ¾ teaspoon of baking powder
- ⅛teaspoon of baking powder
- ¼ cup of milk of your choice, can be milk alternative such as almond milk
- ⅓cup of Nutella
- 2 teaspoons of vanilla extract
- ⅔cups of granulated brown or white sugar
- ¼ cup of rolled oats
- 1 ½ cups of canned chickpeas, drained and rinsed
- ½ cup of chocolate chips

Directions:

1. Preheat your oven to 350 °F and grease an 8" baking tin.
2. In a food processor, add all the ingredients apart from the choc chips. Blitz until well combined and smooth.
3. Add the chocolate chips to the batter, stir with a spatula, and transfer into the baking tin. Spread it evenly by using your spatula.
4. Bake in the oven for 30 minutes. Then remove. Initially, they will look underdone, but this is how they are supposed to be. Allow to cool in the tin, then cover with cling wrap and allow to set overnight in the refrigerator.
5. Once ready, slice and serve.

Calories: 60 kcal per serving.

Tip(s):

1. Cut the sugar if you wish.
2. Swap the chickpeas for white beans instead.
3. Any milk option can be used in this recipe, including coconut milk, but opt for the unsweetened kind.

Cheat Chocolate Cake

Preparation time: 15 minutes

Total cook time: 40 minutes

Serving size: 12 servings

Ingredients for frosting:

- 1 teaspoon of vanilla extract
- 8 oz. of light cool whip, thawed

- 1 cup of low-fat milk
- 1 packet (1.4 oz.) sugar-free instant chocolate pudding

Ingredients for cake:

- 1 cup of water
- 11 oz. of Greek chocolate yogurt
- 15.25 oz. of milk chocolate cake mix, unprepared

Directions:

1. Preheat your oven to 350 °F and grease a 9" by 13" baking tin.
2. In a mixing bowl, combine the cake mix, yogurt, and water until smooth.
3. Transfer the cake mixture into the baking tin and set in the oven to bake for 30 minutes. Once removed from the oven, allow it to cool completely.
4. In a separate mixing bowl, combine the vanilla extract, milk, and instant pudding. Using a hand whisk, combine until smooth and thick.
5. Fold in the cool whip.
6. Spread the frosting mixture over the cooled cake and serve. Add a dash of chocolate sprinkles to the top for extra decadence or opt to grate 70% or more dark chocolate over the top.

Calories: 192 kcal per serving

Tip(s):

1. Use 1% milk as a lower calorie option or use a milk alternative such as coconut or almond milk; unsweetened is always best.

Lemon Cake

Preparation time: 5 minutes

Total cook time: 20 minutes

Serving size: 20 servings

Ingredients:

- Lemon cake mix of choice
- 1 ½ cups of Sprite Zero or sugar-free lemonade

Directions:

1. Preheat your oven to 350 °F
2. Place 20 cupcake liners onto a tray or into a muffin or cupcake tray. Double up so they do not brown.
3. In a mixing bowl, combine the Sprite and cake mix. Stir until the batter is lump-free. Be warned that the batter does fizz; do not worry. It is meant to do this.
4. Spoon the mixture into the liners and place into the oven. Bake for 20 minutes or until baked through.
5. Once ready, remove it from the oven. The cake should be cool before serving.

Calories: 80 kcal per serving.

Tip(s):

1. To add more of a lemon flavor, sprinkle over fresh lemon or lime zest. Or include this in your recipe before baking.

Detox Water

Preparation time: 5 minutes

Total cook time: 5 minutes

Serving size: 4 - 5 cups of water

Ingredients:

- 34 f. oz. of water
- 1 tablespoon of ginger, shredded
- 3 tablespoons of fresh mint
- 1 lemon, sliced and deseeded
- 1 cucumber, sliced

Directions:

1. Prepare all ingredients.
2. Fill a large jar or drinking bottle with the water. Add the remaining ingredients, give it a shake, and drink throughout the day.

Calories: 0

Tip(s):

1. Add more or less of the ingredients depending on your taste.
2. Add 5 to 10sliced strawberries to the detox water.

Cooking Tips

- If you find that you would like certain food items sweeter, add in agave as an alternative, but remember, only if you need to. Avoid sugar as much as possible.
- **Consider investing in a steamer**; try and cook most of your food this way.
- **Opt for low-fat protein**; get this nutrient from by eating pulses and nuts.
- When eating meat, be sure to **remove all the skin and fat** first.

- Try and **eat your fruits and vegetables in their raw form**; cooking often breaks down important nutrients.
- Steer clear of cooking foods such as bell peppers, asparagus, mushrooms, spinach, and carrots; when you do, they lose their most important vitamins that your body can absorb.
- **Cook with extra-virgin olive oil or alternative nut oils.** A low-fat spray-and-cook can also prove useful when cooking certain foods.
- Bland food is boring; **add spices and fresh herbs** to food.
- Eat as many leafy-green vegetables as you can.
- **Keep the skins on fruits and vegetables**; for example, eat apples and pears with the skin on.
- If the weather is cooler, and you find yourself hungry in the mornings, **eat oats**. It will keep you fuller on your fasting days.
- Never weigh your food before cooking; always weigh it after you cook it as this will reflect their true calorie count.
- **Drizzle your salad with extra-virgin olive oil** or alternative dressing such as sesame or avocado oil. The reason for this is because an individual can absorb fat-soluble vitamins easily when tucking into a green salad.
- **Mix your salad up by drizzling lemon juice over it**. The acid found within citrus fruits allows the human body to more easily absorb the iron found in greens such as kale and spinach.
- Pick your pan; the best is a non-stick one.
- Like your milk and cheese? No problem; choose the low-fat options.

- Coffees such as lattes, mochas, and cappuccinos are packed with calories; rather say no to these on fast days.
- **Say no to white, starchy foods.** No more white bread, potato, or pasta. Say yes to low-GI foods and rye, whole-wheat options.

Recipe and Cooking Round-Up

- Stick to natural, healthy, and wholesome foods.
- Eat your fruits and vegetables in their raw form, where you can.
- Say no to processed foods.
- With regards to dairy and meat, keep it lean and low-fat.
- If eating meat, opt for organic, cage-free, and grass-fed.
- If you are looking for something sweet, by all means, try to stick to the dessert recipes mentioned.
- Stay hydrated; drink at least half a gallon of water a day.
- Count your calories.
- Always read the recipe from start to finish before you begin.

Chapter 7: Fasting and Your Lifestyle

"Respect your body. Fuel your body. Challenge your body. Move your body. And most of all, love your body." - Unknown

There is no right or wrong time to start fasting. The best time to start is now, not on Monday, like many of us are inclined to say and do. There is no time like the present.

It is, however, recommended that if you do have any medical conditions, you should discuss this with your doctor.

Prepare yourself, your refrigerator, and pantry. That means have the last few scoops of ice-cream that might be leftover and get rid of anything that might tempt you to *"cheat"* or break your fast.

Fast one a day when you feel as if you can accomplish anything; if you pursue fasting on a day in which you feel half-hearted about it, then it won't work.

A commitment shared with others is also a sure-fire way to stick to your fast. By publicly announcing your wishes to better your life with those closest to you, the more inclined they are to respect the days upon which you fast and make arrangements around your lifestyle.

Do not, on all accounts, decide to begin your fast in the middle of the Christmas season or another holiday period. There are far too many pitfalls during the holiday periods.

Where to From Now?

Now that you have the basics down, the question on most people's lips will be how do I stick with it?

You must understand that like any lifestyle change, it will be difficult. It does get easier with time. You should further understand that while you are saying, "No, thank you" to particular foods one day, you are allowed to return to normal eating the following day. Intermittent fasting is easy to master, unlike many diets that require you to dedicate yourself for months on end, daily.

Deal with your hunger, and though it can make you feel terrible, you must understand you have over enough energy stores in your body to tide you through the phases of uncomfortability.

Know your emotions; as women, we are complex at most times. We eat when happy, we eat when depressed, we eat out of boredom. Come to know your feelings and cut the ties it has with eating.

Reward yourself when you have reached a milestone. Small celebrations keep you motivated. That does not mean you should polish off a box of chocolate but one or two can't hurt.

Fasting is temporary; tomorrow is another day, filled with food, remember, in moderation.

Not everybody is the same. We are all unique and that is also a key to your success. Comparing yourself to somebody else's fasting journey is ok if you use it for motivational purposes, but do not compare the two, as we are all unique.

One Week 16:8 Intermittent Fasting Plan

Day One

7:00 a.m. - One glass of detox water.

7:30 a.m. - Skip your breakfast.

11:00 a.m. - Thai inspired pineapple and chicken salad.

2:00 p.m. - Fruit of your choice, keep to 3.5 and 4 oz.

6:00 p.m. - Spicy bell pepper pilaf.

7:00 p.m. - Stop eating and begin your fast.

Day Two

7:00 a.m. - One glass of detox water.

7:30 a.m. - Skip your breakfast.

11:00 a.m. - Tomato and spinach baked eggs.

2:00 p.m. - Handful of raw, mixed nuts.

6:00 p.m. - Leafy-green soup.

7:00 p.m. - Stop eating and begin your fast.

Day Three

7:00 a.m. - One glass of detox water.

7:30 a.m. - Skip your breakfast.

11:00 a.m. - Grilled chicken salad.

2:00 p.m. - 3.5 to 4 oz. of low-fat yogurt.

6:00 p.m. - Chickpea curry.

7:00 p.m. - Stop eating and begin your fast.

Day Four

7:00 a.m. - One glass of detox water.

7:30 a.m. - Skip your breakfast.

11:00 a.m. - Tuna salad.

2:00 p.m. - Fruit of your choice; keep to 3.5 and 4 oz.

6:00 p.m. - Mixed vegetable and feta tart.

7:00 p.m. - Stop eating and begin your fast.

Day Five

7:00 a.m. - One glass of detox water.

7:30 a.m. - Skip your breakfast.

11 a.m. - Spinach, tomato and ricotta frittata.

2:00 p.m. - Handful of raw, mixed nuts.

6:00 p.m. - Homemade vegetable soup.

7:00 p.m. - Stop eating and begin your fast.

Day Six

7:00 a.m. - One glass of detox water.

7:30 a.m. - Skip your breakfast.

11:00 a.m. - Blueberry porridge.

2:00 p.m. - 3.5 to 4 oz. of low-fat yogurt.

6:00 p.m. - Grilled salmon and leafy-green salad.

7:00 p.m. - Stop eating and begin your fast.

Day Seven

7:00 a.m. - One glass of detox water.

7:30 a.m. - Skip your breakfast.

11:00 a.m. - 1 boiled egg with celery and carrot sticks served with 1 tablespoon of hummus.

2:00 p.m. - Fruit of your choice; keep to 3.5 and 4 oz.

6:00 p.m. - Roast vegetable salad.

7:00 p.m. - Stop eating and begin your fast.

Intermittent Fasting Plan: 2 Days/Week

This plan is based on incorporating two fasting days to your regular, weekly eating pattern. There are six examples of fasting plans that should help support you for three weeks.

Be sure to swap out meals and mix them up so you do not get bored if you wish to follow the below-mentioned meal plan. Remember to also control your portion intake and to be wary of your calories; keep them to between 500 and 600 kcals a day on fast days.

Staying hydrated is also important; keep a bottle of detox water on you to remind you to keep your fluids up. The fasting schedule is 12 hours between meals.

There are three schedules mentioned below to further help you on your way; this is merely a guideline and can prove helpful when planning your week, knowing which days you are fasting versus the days you are eating regularly.

Fast Day One (Week 1)

7:00 a.m. - Blueberry porridge.

7:00 p.m. - Leafy-green soup.

Fast Day Two (Week 1)

7:00 a.m. - One fruit of choice and one boiled egg.

7:00 p.m. - Chickpea curry.

Fast Day One (Week 2)

7:00 a.m. - One cup of low-fat yogurt, one slice of ham, and ½ cup of blueberries.

7:00 p.m. - Basil pesto with whole-wheat durum pasta.

Fast Day Two (Week 2)

7:00 a.m. - One slice of whole-wheat toast with low-fat cream cheese and one fruit of your choice.

7:00 p.m. - Minestrone soup.

Fast Day One (Week 3)

7:00 a.m. - One fruit of choice and one boiled egg.

7:00 p.m. - Roast chicken and leafy-green salad.

Fast Day Two (Week 3)

7:00 a.m. - Blueberry porridge.

7:00 p.m. - Grilled tuna and roast vegetables.

Schedule Options

Option one:

Regular meals: Monday, Tuesday, Wednesday, Thursday, Saturday

Fasting days: Friday and Sunday

Option two:

Regular meals: Tuesday, Wednesday, Friday, Saturday, Sunday

Fasting days: Monday and Thursday

Option three:

Regular meals: Monday, Wednesday, Friday, Saturday and Sunday

Fasting days: Tuesday and Thursday

Fasting and Exercise

Any form of exercise is a universal tool in managing your weight, supporting mental health, and boosting your energy levels.

Exercise can:

- Prevent nagging back pain.
- Increases the levels of good cholesterol in your body and lowers the bad cholesterol.
- Improves memory.
- Uplifts the mood.
- Helps aid and manage weight-loss.
- It lowers blood pressure.
- Eases stress.
- Stabilizes blood sugar levels.

You can fast and exercise at the same time, and you may exercise on the days that you fast too. Your aim is to exercise between 25 and 30 minutes a day. It also does not need to be one solid period dedicated to exercise. **Spread your workouts over three or more days and alternate the type of exercises you do.**

Any amount of time keeping your body moving is good for you; the more, the better.

I am sure that there is a huge sigh of relief to hear this as many struggle to commit to a set workout period; though if you enjoy this, you are welcome to exercise whole-heartedly for the full time.

It is also wise to dedicate two days a week to focus on specific parts of the body, such as the back, arms, and legs.

There are **four facets of exercise you should consider** after the age of 50. They are:

- **Cardio**, which keeps the heart pumping, the blood flowing, and aids in weight-loss.
- **Balance orientated exercise** can prevent stumbles and falls, an incredibly important factor to consider, especially with aging when this becomes more prevalent.
- **Strength training** is wise as it builds and maintains muscle.
- Forms of **stretching exercises**, such as yoga, keep the body limber and pliable, which can help you avoid injury and help recover faster from injury.

Avoid any exercise that can impact your joints, such as skipping, jumping, and pounding. Think less impact.

The following exercises comes highly recommended:

- Golfing
- Tennis
- Yoga
- Thai Chi
- Swimming
- Walking
- Dancing
- Pilates

If any of the above causes discomfort, it would be wise to adjust your schedule and avoid that type of exercise.

Another tip is to **download an app to track your progress**; for those who enjoy walking, an app or smart-watch is the perfect device to count your steps.

Alternative ways to exercise throughout your day:

- Take the stairs.
- Park further away from the entrance of a store.
- Carry your shopping bags one by one into the house than a couple at one time.
- When there are adverts on TV, stand up and walk down the hall or take a quick walk around your yard.
- Collect the laundry from the wash-line piece by piece.

Get started by:

- **Making an exercise schedule for yourself**. Include the days and times you wish to exercise and stick to your plan. Set a reminder on your mobile phone so you do not forget.
- **Exercise in the morning**; you have more energy reserves then!
- **Start gently and then up the level and intensity of your workout** or chosen physical activity, then begin to slow down again as you near the end of the activity or workout.
- **Watch an exercise video** that you can follow in the comfort of your own home.
- **Listen to music** while you exercise; it will keep you motivated.

Yoga Poses to Try at Home

Yoga is a wonderful type of exercise that is beneficial for improving flexibility, mindfulness, and your health. The practice is suited for all ages as it has less impact on muscles and joints than other traditional forms of exercise. The exercises mentioned below are suited and slightly tweaked to accommodate beginners and for women over the age of 50.

Downward facing dog: Grab a chair and face it toward you; make sure the back rests against a wall. Place both of your hands, palms downward, onto the chair. Stand a distance away, feet hip-width apart and firmly planted. Slowly bring your head down between outstretched arms, keeping your spine straight. If you need to bend your knees slightly to relieve the tension you are welcome to.

Hand-to-toe: Stand with your feet firmly planted, keeping the one leg straight, gently raise up the opposite leg to be parallel with the floor. This leg too should be kept straight. Make use of a strap to help guide your leg up and keep it extended.

Tree pose: Standing with your feet planted, raise your leg and place your foot on the inside of the opposite thigh. Gently raise your arms to chest height, and bring your hands together as if in prayer. You may use a chair to support you if needed.

Half lotus: Sit comfortably on a chair with your back and shoulders raised. Cross one leg over the opposite knee. Bring both hands and arms, outstretched and bend forward, attempting to touch the floor with your fingers.

Seated-forward bend: Using a chair, sit comfortably with your back and shoulders kept raised and straight. Extend your legs out in front of you, heels to the ground and toes upward. Gently, keeping your back straight, lean forward and hold your calves. You may lessen the degree at which you do this depending on your comfortability.

Crescent pose: Standing up straight, gently stretch your left leg out behind you, as far as you can. Keep your toes to the ground and your heel up as if you were preparing to launch yourself. Keep your right leg straight and firmly planted on the ground. Gently bring your arms, outstretched over your head. Ensure that your hands are grasping one another. Fingers intertwined with your palms facing upward.

Bridge pose: Lay down on a flat surface. Using a cushion, slide it under your pelvis to support your hips. Bring your legs up and bend your knees, with feet firmly planted on the ground. Keep your arms outstretched alongside you, palms facing upward. Gently use the strength in your shoulders and arms, raise your pelvis up to the ceiling, keep your back straight through this exercise.

Try Meditation

Meditation is becoming more popular by the day in its ability to help manage people's stress levels and help focus the mind. It also teaches us how to be mindful and to become more aware of the impact we have on ourselves and the world around us.

Meditation can go hand-in-hand with intermittent fasting as a way to not only improve your physical health but mental health too.

Stress, after all, is just as bad for you as increased levels of insulin in the body.

It is important when undertaking any challenge, diet or not, to be mentally prepared and have clarity of mind. Being mindful and practicing meditation can help you on your journey.

As we age, we and as women experience menopause; it may lead us to feel hormonal, moody, and depressed. Meditation is one key you can use to help you along through this trying period.

It comes with a range of benefits, which include:

- Extends attention span.
- Reduces age-related memory loss.
- Improves sleep.
- Moderates blood pressure
- Controls mental illness such as anxiety and depression.
- Manages stress.

How to practice mindful meditation using the following steps:

1. Find a quiet and comfortable place to meditate; this can be indoors or outdoors, wherever you are most at ease. You may either sit on a chair with your hands folded on your lap or you may proceed to lay down. Whatever pose you choose to hold, make sure it is one you wish to hold; fidgeting will only break your focus.

2. When you have chosen your space, make sure there are no distractions or put these away or turn, for example, your phone off.

3. Begin your meditation practice by closing your eyes and allowing your thoughts to come to a rest. Do not try and wish these thoughts away or interject them; let them come and go at their time and pace.

4. Try to get to a moment where all you are doing is focusing on the present moment.

5. Slowly become aware of your breath, the way it affects your body, raising your chest and lowering your chest. Feel the flow of air running up into your nose and out again. Focus on how each breath is different.

6. Allow all thoughts to come and go, no matter if they are happy or upsetting ones. These thoughts do not

define you. If you find yourself going along with a particular thought, return your attention to your breath. Use your breath as a weight for when you find yourself trailing off.

7. Do not be hard on yourself; meditation comes with time, patience, and practice.

8. Stay this way for however long you feel is comfortable.

9. When you wish to exit your meditation, stay seated or lying down for another minute or two before standing up.

Fasting Round-Up, Tips to Keep You Focused

Here is a round-up of ways in which you can make the lifestyle work for you:

- Most importantly, when you have reached a milestone, **congratulate yourself**.

- **Weight-loss is not a given but will happen over time**. There will be days when the scale remains unchanged, and there will be days when the scale will drop.

- Before you start, **weigh yourself, take your measurements, and know your BMI**.

- **Keep a journal**, and track your progress.

- **Keep your fluids up** throughout the day.

- **Prepare your meals the day before** if you can; that way you are inclined to stick to your fast days better.

- **Rope in a few friends** who are eager to also make a lifestyle change.

- **Read all food packaging** for those hidden calories, sugars, and preservatives. There is a range of apps that can tell you exactly how many calories are in items of food.

- **Keep active**; a busy mind is less inclined to send you to the kitchen for a bite to eat.

- **Chew gum**, it aids digestion, and takes your mind off feeling hungry and the time.

- **Meditate** for better health and moods.

- **Stick to healthy foods** and leave the "*bad*" ones alone.

- **Alternate your fast days**; two consecutive days in a row can prove difficult and hard to stick with.

- **Be consistent when it comes to your fasting days**; your hard work will pay off.

Chapter 8: To Future Health

"Next time you think of beautiful things, don't forget to count yourself in!" - Anonymous

One of the most important things you can do for your longevity aside from intermittent fasting and consuming whole foods outside of fasting and exercising are the health checks you should pursue at a health facility or your local doctor's office.

Health Checks for Women

The following are **important tests that should be conducted** to know exactly where you stand regarding your health and address any concerns that might be noted by either yourself or the doctor.

Cholesterol

Cholesterol is present in all our cells. The 20% of cholesterol in our body's comes from the food we consume; the other 80% is what your body creates. **High cholesterol counts can cause blockages within the arteries** and can cause you to develop a risk for stroke or suffer a heart attack. You should have yours tested every three years. Cholesterol is subdivided into three categories: total cholesterol, the good and bad cholesterol. Total levels of cholesterol should be lower than 200 milligrams per deciliter.

Low-density lipoproteins (LDL) or "bad" cholesterol should be less than 100 mg/dl. If your figures read between 200 and 239 mg/dl, it is considered ok if you have no health history that is of concern; however, if heart disease is prevalent in your family, this figure would be concerning. Between 130 and 159 mg/dl is what is considered borderline high, 160 to 189 mg/dl is high, and a reading of 190 mg/dl is very, very high and seen as dangerous.

The levels of your good cholesterol or HDL (high-density lipoproteins) should be even higher than the LDL count.

Blood Pressure
High blood pressure can influence your heart negatively and place unwanted stress on the heart and arteries. High blood pressure may result in suffering from kidney disease, stroke, or a heart attack. Blood pressure is divided into two categories: your systolic pressure and your diastolic pressure.

You will notice when your blood pressure is recorded, it will show up as two sets of numbers that are separated; these are the different pressures. A systolic pressure of over 140 is concerning in patients that are over 50 years old. Diastolic pressure of 90 and under is deemed ok.

Blood Sugar Levels
Blood tests are useful in testing for pre-diabetes or diabetes. Blood sugar levels are impacted by your diet, amount of physical activity you do, weight, and level of insulin resistance. Other factors that are important to

mention are if you have a family with a history of diabetes too.

Those who suffer from low blood sugar can fall into a coma or suffer a seizure, and those who have high levels of blood sugar can develop diabetes and further heart complications.

The two tests for you to consider are the fasting blood sugar test and hemoglobin A1C test.

The following will provide a guideline as to what your blood sugar levels should look like on a normal scale.

Diabetic	Pre-diabetic	Regular
Higher than or equivalent to 126 mg/dl	Between 110 and 125 mg/dl	Below 100 mg/dl
Higher than or equivalent to 6.5%	Between 5.7 and 6.4%	Below 5.7%

Further Testing

Further tests to conduct can include:

- Urine tests

- Blood tests

- Pap smears and pelvic health tests

- Breast health checks such as ultrasound or mammograms

- Eye tests

- A visit to the dentist

- Check-in with your dermatologist regarding marks and moles on your body

Face Value

The same we undertake to look after our body through the exercise, we should do the same for our face. The face does lose elasticity and tone when aging, and by exercising it, you can stave off fine lines and wrinkles and reduce those that have already traced their way around areas of your face.

The forehead holds the finest lines and wrinkles, so to help simulate this area, try the following exercise:

Close your eyes, and using your fingertips, make small circular movements on your forehead. Use light pressure and continue to do this for five minutes. Or try pressing the palm against the forehead and then attempt to move our head downward. Practice this exercise for five minutes too.

The Holistic Approach

Let us face it, looking after our bodies, health, and skin can be expensive, but it doesn't have to be. Intermittent fasting is an affordable approach to dieting; walking in the neighborhood park or down the beach is free. What about skincare? Skincare needn't carry a price tag too.

A combination of a few ingredients found within your pantry can go a long way in your salad but can be used to create facial and body scrubs and make for great ingredients to add into your bath.

Face Masks

Avo and oats face mask: ½ avocado, 1 tablespoon of rolled oats, ground up finely, 1 teaspoon of lemon juice, 1 teaspoon of coconut oil, 1 tablespoon of honey, and 2 drops of essential oil such as lavender or chamomile. Mash up all the ingredients in a bowl, and apply to your face. Allow the mask to rest upon your face for 20 minutes before washing it off with warm water. Store the rest in an airtight container in the refrigerator and use it within the next day as it makes four servings.

Banana mask: 5 tablespoons of rolled oats, ground up finely, 1 ripe banana, and 1 tablespoon of honey. Mash the banana and stir in the oats and honey. Stir once more to combine and then apply to your face for 20 minutes. Rinse off with warm water.

Lemon face mask: 2 tablespoons baking soda, 1 teaspoon of honey, ½ a tablespoon of fresh lemon juice, and 1 teaspoon of water. Combine in a bowl. Apply to your skin and allow to rest for 15 minutes. Rinse off with warm water.

Body Scrubs

Coconut and sugar scrub: 10 drops of essential oil of your choice (rose works well), 2 oz. of granulated brown sugar, and 2 fl. oz. of coconut oil. Combine and apply to the entire body, focusing on the rough areas such as elbows and feet. Climb into the shower or bath and rinse off. Bathing is recommended as the scrub will melt off your body and dissolve in the bath; lay in the bath for however long you wish.

Bath Soak Recipes

Detox bath soak: 10 drops of essential oil (mint works well), 2 oz. of Himalayan salt, 2 oz. of bicarbonate soda, 2 oz. of Epsom salt, and 3 oz. of apple cider vinegar. Combine these in a heat proof container, fill with boiling water, and allow to dissolve; then add it into your bath. Soak for between 20 to 30 minutes.

To Future Health Round-Up

- Make use of sugar in your beauty products. It hydrates the skin.

- Almond oil is rich in vitamins A, B, and E. It is good for those who have irritable skin.

- Oats contain vitamin E, a rich antioxidant, and it makes for a great exfoliant.

- Honey works as an antiseptic and is helpful to include in masks and scrubs because it limits breakouts.

- Lemon is also antiseptic and can be used just as it is on your hair to treat hair fall and dandruff.

- Egg repairs skin tissues that have been damaged and tones the skin. For aged skin, it keeps the skin elastic, and for younger skin, it is known to tighten pores.

- Avocado and the vitamins it contains such as unsaturated oils can easily be absorbed through the skin and is perfect to add to your skin with nothing else.

- Bananas are rich in B6 and vitamin C, which maintain the elasticity of the skin.

Conclusion

"Just because you don't see results after a day or even a week, don't give up. You may not see changes, but every smart choice you make is affecting you in ways you'd never imagine." - Julia Farver

Over time you will slowly begin to see the results that fasting has on your body. Understand that disappointments also arise, but whatever you do, do not give up!

Gradually over time, you will notice the scale drop and your clothes will begin to sit on you less tightly.

For the health-conscious, fasting over time will also lower your cholesterol levels, which are pivotal in avoiding heart complications and disease. Plus, it can help prevent developing pre-diabetes.

As we age, our energy levels begin to dwindle; however, the rewards of fasting should, one all accounts, begin to put more pep in your step. For those who have stroppy bowels, it should begin to regulate them too.

Fasting will change the way you eat and look at fat altogether. Soon you will find yourself saying "no" to certain foods even on days you do not find yourself fasting. This is not because you do not want to reward or treat yourself but because you do not feel like you need to eat a slice of chocolate cake. You will also learn to understand what a feeling of satisfaction feels like versus stuffed to the brim.

Intermittent fasting allows us to spot check our diet and change our attitude long-term. Say hello to longevity, clarity, improved health, weight-loss, and fewer aches and pains.

Sounds worth it, doesn't it? Time to get started….

I am happy to have shared this book with you and I really hope you enjoyed it. Please let me know your thoughts by leaving a short review on Amazon. Thanks again!

References

[1] Gunnars, K. (2017, June 4). What Is Intermittent Fasting? Explained in Human

Terms. Retrieved from

https://www.healthline.com/nutrition/what-is-intermittent-fasting

[2] Thompson, D. (2019, December 26). 'Intermittent Fasting' Diet Could Boost Your

Health. Retrieved from

https://www.webmd.com/diet/news/20191226/intermittent-fasting-diet-could-boost-your-health#1

[3] Lopez-Jimenez, F. (2019, January 9). Wondering about fasting and heart health?

Retrieved from

https://www.mayoclinic.org/diseases-conditions/heart-disease/expert-answers/fasting-diet/faq-20058334?mc_id=us&utm_source=newsnetwork&utm_medium=l&utm_content=content&utm_campaign=mayoclinic&geo=national&placementsite=enterprise&cauid=100721&_ga=2.3021680.1594255446.1582146435-463905821.1582146435

[4] Know Your Risk for Heart Disease. (2019, December 10). Retrieved from

https://www.cdc.gov/heartdisease/risk_factors.htm

[5] Gunnars, K. (2018, July 25). Intermittent Fasting 101 – The Ultimate Beginner's

Guide. Retrieved from

https://www.healthline.com/nutrition/intermittent-fasting-guide#weight-loss

[6] Trafton, A. (2018, May 3). Fasting boosts stem cells' regenerative capacity. Retrieved

from http://news.mit.edu/2018/fasting-boosts-stem-cells-regenerative-capacity-0503

[7] Dockrill, P. (n.d.). Fasting For Just 24 Hours Boosts The Regeneration of Stem Cells,

Study Finds. Retrieved from

https://www.sciencealert.com/fasting-for-just-24-hours-boosts-the-regeneration-of-stem-cells-study-finds-intestine-longevity

[8] Sol, M. V. (2018, November 21). Fasting for 72 Hours Can Reset Your Entire

Immune System. Retrieved from

https://thesource.com/2018/11/21/fasting-for-72-hours-can-reset-your-entire-immune-system/

[9] Fung, J. (2019, September 11). Fasting and growth hormone. Retrieved from

https://www.dietdoctor.com/fasting-and-growth-hormone

[10] Fung, J. (2018, September 14). How fasting affects your physiology and hormones.

Retrieved from

https://www.dietdoctor.com/fasting-affects-physiology-hormones

[11] Fung, J. (2018, September 14). How fasting affects your physiology and hormones.

Retrieved from

https://www.dietdoctor.com/fasting-affects-physiology-hormones

[12] Santos-Longhurst, A. (2017, February 27). Type 2 Diabetes Statistics and Facts.

Healthline. https://www.healthline.com/health/type-2-diabetes/statistics

[13] Wondering about fasting and heart health? (2019, January 9). Retrieved from

https://www.mayoclinic.org/diseases-conditions/heart-disease/expert-answers/fasting-diet/faq-20058334

[14] Regular fasting could lead to longer, healthier life. (n.d.). Retrieved from

https://www.heart.org/en/news/2019/11/25/regular-fasting-could-lead-to-longer-healthier-life

[15] Tello, M. (2020, February 10). Intermittent fasting: Surprising update. Retrieved

from https://www.health.harvard.edu/blog/intermittent-fasting-surprising-update-2018062914156

[16] Arora, G. (2019, November 20). Intermittent Fasting And Circadian Rhythm: 10

Tips To Make Intermittent Fasting Work For You. Retrieved from

https://www.ndtv.com/health/intermittent-fasting-and-circadian-rhythm-10-tips-to-bring-fasting-in-line-with-your-bodys-biologica-2135654

[17] Circadian Rhythms. (n.d.). Retrieved from

https://www.nigms.nih.gov/education/pages/factsheet_circadianrhythms.aspx

[18] Lindberg, S. (2018, August 23). Autophagy: Definition, Diet, Fasting, Cancer,

Benefits, and More. Healthline. https://www.healthline.com/health/autophagy

[19] Fung, J. (2019, September 10). How to Renew Your Body: Fasting and Autophagy.

Retrieved from https://www.dietdoctor.com/renew-body-fasting-autophagy

[20] Eske, J. (2019, January 14). Fasting and cancer: Benefits and effects. Retrieved

from

https://www.medicalnewstoday.com/articles/324169

[21] Griffith, T. (2018, September 29). Fasting and Cancer: The Science Behind This

Treatment Method. Retrieved from

https://www.healthline.com/health/fasting-and-cancer#research

[22] Fung, J. (2016, January 28). Intermittent Fasting for Beginners. Retrieved from

https://www.dietdoctor.com/intermittent-fasting#weightloss

[23] Can Intermittent Fasting Help Treat Depression? (2019, January 8). Retrieved

from

https://www.psychcongress.com/article/can-intermittent-fasting-help-treat-depression

[24] Facts & Statistics. (n.d.). Retrieved from

https://adaa.org/about-adaa/press-room/facts-statistics

[25] How Does Fasting Affect the Brain? (n.d.). Retrieved from

https://www.brainfacts.org/thinking-sensing-and-behaving/diet-and-lifestyle/2018/how-does-fasting-affect-the-brain-071318

[26] Facts and Figures. (n.d.). Retrieved from

https://www.alz.org/alzheimers-dementia/facts-figures

[27] Jorgenson. (2020, February 22). The Growing Science Behind a Fasting Treatment

for Alzheimer's. Retrieved from

https://www.discovermagazine.com/health/the-growing-science-behind-a-fasting-treatment-for-alzheimers

[28] Seana. (1968, January 1). Can fasting give you more energy? Retrieved from

https://www.freeletics.com/en/blog/posts/intermittent-fasting/

[29] Can fasting lead to better skin? (n.d.). Retrieved from

https://www.msn.com/en-us/health/medical/can-fasting-lead-to-better-skin/ar-AAGRVaq

[30] Health24: Whoops We've Gone into Cardiac Arrest. (n.d.). Health Information,

News & Lifestyle Tips | Health24.

https://www.health24.com/Lifestyle/aging-well/News/How-your-body-changes-after-50-20150203

[31] Migala, B. J., Upham, B., Migala, J., & Millard, E. (n.d.). 6 Types of Intermittent

Fasting: Which Is Best for You?: Everyday Health. Retrieved from

https://www.everydayhealth.com/diet-nutrition/diet/types-intermittent-fasting-which-best-you/

[32] Free BMI Calculator - Calculate Your Body Mass Index. (n.d.). Retrieved from

https://bmicalculatorusa.com/

6 Ways to Practice Mindful Eating. (2019, November 19). Retrieved from

https://www.mindful.org/6-ways-practice-mindful-eating/

9 Homemade Face Mask Recipes That Actually Work. (n.d.). Retrieved from

https://www.readersdigest.ca/health/beauty/homemade-facial-masks-recipes/

About Glycemic Index. (n.d.). Retrieved from

https://www.gisymbol.com/about-glycemic-index/

Axe, J. (2017, June 19). The 5 Most Common Fasting Mistakes-And How to Fix Them.

Retrieved from

https://observer.com/2017/06/most-common-intermittent-fasting-mistakes/

Body Changes After 50: How Much Can You Control? (2016, December 20). Next

Avenue. https://www.nextavenue.org/body-changes-50-control/

Brohl, P. (2019, November 14). 11 Low-Calorie Green Smoothie Recipes Under 100

Calories. Retrieved from

https://vibranthappyhealthy.com/low-calorie-smoothies

Buenfeld, S. (2015, February 1). Porridge with blueberry compote. Retrieved from

https://www.bbcgoodfood.com/recipes/porridge-blueberry-compote

Cadogan, M. (2009, May 1). Asparagus soldiers with a soft-boiled egg. Retrieved from

https://www.bbcgoodfood.com/recipes/asparagus-soldiers-soft-boiled-egg

Changes in Hormone Levels. (n.d.). Retrieved from

https://www.menopause.org/for-women/sexual-health-menopause-online/changes-at-midlife/changes-in-hormone-levels

Chickpea, tomato & spinach curry. (2011, May 1). Retrieved from

https://www.bbcgoodfood.com/recipes/chickpea-tomato-spinach-curry

Contraindications of Fasting. (n.d.). Retrieved from

http://timaltman.com.au/contraindications-of-fasting/

Cook, S. (2012, November 1). Creamy tomato soup. Retrieved from https://www.bbcgoodfood.com/recipes/creamy-tomato-soup

Corrett, N. (2015, January 1). Broccoli and kale green soup. Retrieved from

https://www.bbcgoodfood.com/recipes/alkalising-green-soup

Coyle, D. (2017, November 7). A Beginner's Guide to the Low-Glycemic Diet. Retrieved

from https://www.healthline.com/nutrition/low-glycemic-diet#section8

Diaz, C. (2016). *The Longevity Book: The Biology of Resilience Privilege of Time and*

the New. Harper Collins UK.

Donovan, J. (n.d.). How to Get the Vitamins You Need as You Age. Retrieved from

https://www.webmd.com/healthy-aging/over-50-nutrition-17/vitamin-essentials-as-we-age

Fasting Apps: 6 Best Intermittent Fasting Apps in 2020. (2020, January 23). Retrieved

from https://www.spaceotechnologies.com/best-intermittent-fasting-apps-in-2020/

Fasting benefits, tips, contraindications, & "feat-famine" cycling. (2017, November 21).

Retrieved from

http://kinetik-fitness.com/show-all/1287/fasting-benefits-tips-contraindications-feast-famine-cycling/

Fletcher, J. (2020, January 5). Cholesterol levels by age: Differences and

recommendations. Retrieved from

https://www.medicalnewstoday.com/articles/315900#recommended-levels

Food, G. (2011, October 1). Baked eggs with spinach & tomato. Retrieved from

   https://www.bbcgoodfood.com/recipes/baked-eggs-spinach-tomato

Frost, S., Davidson, H., & Rose, A. (2014). *Deliciously healthy: for your mind, body &*

   soul. London: Kyle Books

Fung, J. (2016, January 28). Intermittent Fasting for Beginners. Retrieved from

   https://www.dietdoctor.com/intermittent-fasting

Fung, J. (2018, September 14). How fasting affects your physiology and hormones.

   Retrieved from

   https://www.dietdoctor.com/fasting-affects-physiology-hormones

Funke, L. (2019, June 9). DIY Oatmeal Avocado Face Mask. Retrieved from

   https://fitfoodiefinds.com/diy-oatmeal-avocado-face-mask/

Funston, L. (2020, February 26). Avocado Egg Boats Make Your Mornings Dreamy.

   Retrieved from

   https://www.delish.com/cooking/recipe-ideas/recipes/a45382/avocado-egg-boats-recipe/

Glycemic Index Chart: GI Ratings for Hundreds of Foods. (2019, July 1). Retrieved from

   https://universityhealthnews.com/daily/nutrition/glycemic-index-chart/

Gould, S. (2017, May 10). 6 charts that show how much more Americans eat than they

   used to. Retrieved from

https://www.businessinsider.com/daily-calories-americans-eat-increase-2016-07/?r=AU&IR=T

Gunnars, K. (2017, August 1). Processed foods: Health risks and dangers. Retrieved

from
https://www.medicalnewstoday.com/articles/318630

Ham & beetroot salad bowl. (2007, August 1). Retrieved from

https://www.bbcgoodfood.com/recipes/ham-beetroot-salad-bowl

Harvard Health Publishing. (n.d.). Women--especially older women--need to pay more

attention to blood pressure, reports the Harvard Women's Health Watch.

Retrieved from

https://www.health.harvard.edu/press_releases/women-especially-older-women-need-to-pay-more-attention-to-blood-pressure

Healthy Carrot Cake Cupcakes - Low-Calorie, Low-Fat! (2019, April 11). Retrieved from

https://chocolatecoveredkatie.com/2015/04/01/healthy-carrot-cake-cupcakes/comment-page-2/

Homepage. (2019, October 9). Retrieved from https://www.fitwirr.com/

Intermittent Fasting – Questions & Answers with Dr. Fung. (2019, September 10).

Retrieved from

https://www.dietdoctor.com/intermittent-fasting/questions-and-answers#diet

Intermittent Fasting for Weight Loss: How It Works and How to Get Started. (2019,

December 27). Retrieved from

https://www.bulletproof.com/diet/intermittent-fasting/intermittent-fasting-weight-loss/

Kamb, S. (2020, January 1). Intermittent Fasting For Beginners: Should You Skip

>   Breakfast? Retrieved from

>   https://www.nerdfitness.com/blog/a-beginners-guide-to-intermittent-fasting/#tips_for_intermittent_fasting

Kirkpatrick, B., & Johnstone, A. (2018). *Healthy hormones: a practical guide to*

>   *balancing your hormones*. Sydney: Murdoch Books.

Kiser, T. (2018, July 1). Healthy Frozen Strawberry Dessert. Retrieved from

>   https://www.foodfaithfitness.com/strawberry-dessert-frozen/

Kiser, T. (2019, September 26). Orange Carrot Smoothie with Ginger. Retrieved from

>   https://www.foodfaithfitness.com/orange-carrot-smoothie-with-ginger/

Leonard, J. (2020, January 9). 7 ways to do intermittent fasting: Best methods and

>   quick tips. Retrieved from

>   https://www.medicalnewstoday.com/articles/322293#tips-for-maintaining-intermittent-fasting

Lewis, E. (2011, January 1). Spiced pepper pilafs. Retrieved from

>   https://www.bbcgoodfood.com/recipes/spiced-pepper-pilafs

Low calorie lemon cupcakes - Skinny cupcakes recipe. (2018, August 23). Retrieved

>   from   https://www.eatingonadime.com/low-calorie-lemon-cupcakes-only-80-calories/

Marie, K., Thomas, M., & Flynn, J. A. (2016). *Slow ageing guide to skin rejuvenation:*

>   *learn, understand, select, proven treatments*. Ingleburn, NSW: Health Informed.

Merkley, K. (2019, August 23). Watermelon Smoothie - Under 100 Calories. Retrieved

   from https://lilluna.com/watermelon-smoothie/

Moisturizing Banana Facial Mask. (2003, January 7). Retrieved from

   https://www.food.com/recipe/moisturizing-banana-facial-mask-50129

Moroccan chickpea soup. (2005, February 1). Retrieved from

   https://www.bbcgoodfood.com/recipes/moroccan-chickpea-soup-0

Mosley, M., & Spencer, M. (2013). *The fast diet: the simple secret of intermittent*

   fasting: lose weight, stay healthy, live longer. London: SB.

Nathalie Rhone, MS, RDN, CDN. (n.d.). Top 10 Anti-Aging Foods for Skin, Brain,

   Muscle, and Gut Health. Healthline.

   https://www.healthline.com/health/food-nutrition/anti-aging-foods#6

Netherton, L. (2013, December 1). Griddled vegetable & feta tart. Retrieved from

   https://www.bbcgoodfood.com/recipes/griddled-vegetable-feta-tart

Netherton, L. (2014, March 1). Spiced chicken & pineapple salad. Retrieved from

   https://www.bbcgoodfood.com/recipes/spiced-chicken-pineapple-salad

Nice, M. (2016, February 1). Roasted spiced cauliflower. Retrieved from

   https://www.bbcgoodfood.com/recipes/roasted-spiced-cauliflower

Nutella Chocolate Chip Blondies. (2016, March 21). Retrieved from https://chocolatecoveredkatie.com/2014/09/23/nutella-chocolate-chip-blondies/

Palmer, N. (2020, January 27). How to make an omelette. Retrieved from

https://www.goodtoknow.co.uk/food/how-to/how-to-make-an-omelette-294964

Primeau, A. S. B. (2019, March 12). Intermittent Fasting and Cancer. Retrieved from

https://www.cancertherapyadvisor.com/home/tools/fact-sheets/intermittent-fasting-and-cancer/2/

Quinn, S. (2018, March 22). Skinny Pineapple Cheesecake Bars. Retrieved from

https://www.delish.com/cooking/recipe-ideas/recipes/a45560/skinny-pineapple-cheesecake-bars-recipe/

Red lentil & sweet potato pâté. (2012, February 1). Retrieved from

https://www.bbcgoodfood.com/recipes/red-lentil-sweet-potato-pate

Ricotta, tomato & spinach frittata. (2011, April 1). Retrieved from

https://www.bbcgoodfood.com/recipes/ricotta-tomato-spinach-frittata

Schend, J. (2020, February 20). 15 Foods That Boost the Immune System. Retrieved

from

https://www.healthline.com/health/food-nutrition/foods-that-boost-the-immune-system#broccoli

Sharp, A. (2019, May 31). The Most Common Mistakes People Make While Intermittent

Fasting. Retrieved from

https://greatist.com/eat/intermittent-fasting-mistakes#1

Sinkus, T. (2020, February 24). A Beginner's Guide to Intermittent Fasting Daily Plan &

Schedule (Updated). Retrieved from

https://21dayhero.com/intermittent-fasting-daily-plan/

Skinny Blueberry Lemon Smoothie. (2018, June 8). Retrieved from

https://happyhealthymama.com/skinny-blueberry-lemon-smoothie.html

Skinny Chocolate Cake. (2020, January 8). Retrieved from

https://togetherasfamily.com/skinny-chocolate-cake/

Stuffed marrow bake. (2011, September 1). Retrieved from

https://www.bbcgoodfood.com/recipes/stuffed-marrow-bake

The best foods for mental health. (n.d.). Retrieved from

https://headspace.org.au/blog/the-best-foods-for-mental-health/

Thomas, M. C. (2017). *The longevity list.* Chatswood, Australia: Exisle Publishing Pty

Ltd.

Thorpe, M. (2017, July 5). 12 Science-Based Benefits of Meditation. Retrieved from

https://www.healthline.com/nutrition/12-benefits-of-meditation#section1

Urinary Incontinence in Women Symptoms, Causes & Treatment. (2019, December 20).

Retrieved from

https://www.medicinenet.com/urinary_incontinence_in_women/article.htm

Varady, K., & Gottlieb, B. (2014). *The every other day diet: the only fasting diet proven*

by science. London: Yellow Kite.

Wake-Up Smoothie. (n.d.). Retrieved from

http://www.eatingwell.com/recipe/248810/wake-up-smoothie/

Watermelon, prawn & avocado salad. (2010, August 1). Retrieved from

https://www.bbcgoodfood.com/recipes/watermelon-prawn-avocado-salad

Wong, C. (2020, February 3). Mindfulness Meditation - How Do I Do It? Retrieved from

https://www.verywellmind.com/mindfulness-meditation-88369

Working Out When You're Over 50. (n.d.). Retrieved from

https://www.webmd.com/fitness-exercise/ss/slideshow-exercise-after-age-50

Yoga Over 50 - 14 Yoga Poses That You Can Do At Any Age. (n.d.). Retrieved from

https://lotsofyoga.com/blogs/yoga-tips/yoga-over-50-best-yoga-poses

Your Body in Your 50s: Hair, Skin, Brain Health, and More. (n.d.). Retrieved from

https://www.webmd.com/healthy-aging/ss/slideshow-what-to-expect-in-your-50s

Zelman, K. M. (2008, May 8). Why Drink More Water? See 6 Health Benefits of Water.

Retrieved from

https://www.webmd.com/diet/features/6-reasons-to-drink-water#2

CPSIA information can be obtained
at www.ICGtesting.com
Printed in the USA
LVHW081255190121
676879LV00035B/260